Women's Health

Editors

DIANE M. HARPER
EMILY M. GODFREY

PRIMARY CARE:
CLINICS IN OFFICE PRACTICE

www.primarycare.theclinics.com

Consulting Editor
JOEL J. HEIDELBAUGH

December 2018 • Volume 45 • Number 4

ELSEVIER

1600 John F. Kennedy Boulevard • Suite 1800 • Philadelphia, Pennsylvania, 19103-2899

http://www.theclinics.com

PRIMARY CARE: CLINICS IN OFFICE PRACTICE Volume 45, Number 4
December 2018 ISSN 0095-4543, ISBN-13: 978-0-323-61380-4

Editor: Jessica McCool
Developmental Editor: Laura Fisher

Primary Care: Clinics in Office Practice (ISSN: 0095-4543) is published quarterly by Elsevier Inc., 360 Park Avenue South, New York, NY 10010-1710. Months of issue are March, June, September, and December. Periodicals postage paid at New York, NY and additional mailing offices. Subscription prices are $237.00 per year (US individuals), $474.00 (US institutions), $100.00 (US students), $289.00 (Canadian individuals), $536.00 (Canadian institutions), $175.00 (Canadian students), $355.00 (international individuals), $536.00 (international institutions), and $175.00 (international students). Foreign air speed delivery is included in all *Clinics* subscription prices. All prices are subject to change without notice. POSTMASTER: Send address changes to *Primary Care: Clinics in Office Practice*, Elsevier Periodicals Customer Service, 11830 Westline Industrial Drive, St. Louis, MO 63146. Customer Service Health Sciences Division, Subscription Customer Service, 3251 Riverport Lane, Maryland Heights, MO 63043. **Customer Service: 1-800-654-2452 (U.S. and Canada); 314-447-8871 (outside U.S. and Canada). Fax: 314-447-8029. E-mail: journalscustomerservice-usa@elsevier.com (for print support); journalsonlinesupport-usa@elsevier.com (for online support).**

Reprints. For copies of 100 or more, of articles in this publication, please contact the Commercial Reprints Department, Elsevier Inc., 360 Park Avenue South, New York, NY 10010-1710. Tel. 212-633-3874; Fax: 212-633-3820; E-mail: reprints@elsevier.com.

Primary Care: Clinics in Office Practice is covered in *MEDLINE/PubMed (Index Medicus)* and *EMBASE/ Excerpta Medica, Current Contents/Clinical Medicine,* and *ISI/BIOMED.*

Contributors

CONSULTING EDITOR

JOEL J. HEIDELBAUGH, MD, FAAFP, FACG
Clinical Professor, Departments of Family Medicine and Urology, University of Michigan Medical School, Ann Arbor, Michigan

EDITORS

DIANE M. HARPER, MD, MPH, MS
Professor and Chair, Department of Family and Geriatric Medicine, University of Louisville School of Medicine, Louisville, Kentucky

EMILY M. GODFREY, MD, MPH
Associate Professor, Family Medicine and Obstetrics and Gynecology, University of Washington, Seattle, Washington

AUTHORS

DEANNA ADKINS, MD
Assistant Professor of Pediatrics, Duke Child and Adolescent Gender Care, Duke University Health System, Durham, North Carolina

JENNIFER R. AMICO, MD, MPH
Assistant Professor, Department of Family Medicine and Community Health, Rutgers Robert Wood Johnson Medical School, New Brunswick, New Jersey

MICHELLE CANGIANO, MD
Physician Site Leader, Assistant Professor, Department of Family Medicine, The Robert Larner, M.D. College of Medicine, University of Vermont, Burlington, Vermont

JENNIFER CHANG, MD
Assistant Professor, Department of Family Medicine, F. Edward Hebert School of Medicine, Uniformed Services University of the Health Sciences, Bethesda, Maryland

TERRI L. CHENG, MD
Assistant Professor, Department of Family Medicine and Public Health, University of California, San Diego, San Diego, California

STEPHANIE A. COCKRELL, LMSW, MSW
Senior Program Manager for Research, Department of Family and Community Medicine, The University of New Mexico, Albuquerque, New Mexico

MELANIE CAMEJO COFFIGNY, JD
Undergraduate Student, Duke University, Durham, North Carolina

TIFFANY COVAS, MD, MPH
Associate Professor, Department of Community and Family Medicine, Duke University Health System, Durham, North Carolina

JENNIFER P. DAILY, MD, CAQSM
Primary Care Sports Medicine Fellowship, KentuckyOne Health, Assistant Professor, Department of Family and Geriatric Medicine, Centers for Primary Care, University of Louisville, Louisville, Kentucky

JESSICA DALBY, MD
Assistant Professor, Department of Family Medicine and Community Health, University of Wisconsin-Madison School of Medicine and Public Health, University of Wisconsin-Madison, Madison, Wisconsin

JAIVIDHYA DASARATHY, MD, FAAFP
Director of Research Education, Associate Professor, Department of Family Medicine, MetroHealth Medical Center, Case Western Reserve University, Cleveland, Ohio

MICHELLE M. DE SOUZA, MD, FACS
Assistant Professor, Department of Plastic Surgery, University of Kansas School of Medicine, Kansas City, Kansas

EMILY M. GODFREY, MD, MPH
Associate Professor, Family Medicine and Obstetrics and Gynecology, University of Washington, Seattle, Washington

SAMUEL N. GRIEF, MD, FCFP, FAAFP
Associate Professor, Department of Family Medicine, The University of Illinois at Chicago, Chicago, Illinois

ADRIENNE HAMPTON, MD
Assistant Professor, Department of Family Medicine and Community Health, University of Wisconsin-Madison School of Medicine and Public Health, University of Wisconsin-Madison, Madison, Wisconsin

GEORGE D. HARRIS, MD, MS
Chair, Professor, Primary Care, Medical Director, UHP, West Virginia University Eastern Division, Martinsburg, West Virginia

SHARON HULL, MD, MPH
Professor, Department of Community and Family Medicine, Associate Certified Coach, ICF, Director, Duke University School of Medicine Executive Coaching Program, Duke University School of Medicine, Durham, North Carolina

JAMAL ISLAM, MD, MS
Associate Professor, Program Director, Family Medicine Residency, University of Texas Medical Branch, Galveston, Texas

ALICIA A. JACOBS, MD
Vice Chair of Clinical Operations, Associate Professor, Department of Family Medicine, The Robert Larner, M.D. College of Medicine at the University of Vermont, Burlington, Vermont

ANDREA D. JEWELL, MD
Assistant Professor, Department of Obstetrics and Gynecology, University of Kansas School of Medicine, Kansas City, Kansas

HALLIE LABRADOR, MD, MS
Associate Director, Primary Care Sports Medicine Fellowship, NorthShore University HealthSystem, Clinician Educator, The University of Chicago Pritzker School of Medicine, Chicago, Illinois

JESSICA LAPINSKI, DO
Duke University Resident Physician, Department of Community and Family Medicine, Duke University Health System, Duke University, Durham, North Carolina

BETHANY PANCHAL, MD
Assistant Professor, Department of Family Medicine, The Ohio State University, Columbus, Ohio

ALISHA N. PARADA, MD, FACP
Assistant Professor, Department of Internal Medicine, Vice Chair of Diversity and Inclusion, The University of New Mexico School of Medicine, UNM Health Sciences Center, Albuquerque, New Mexico

JENNIFER M. PERKINS, MD, MBA
Division of Diabetes, Endocrinology, and Metabolism, Associate Professor, Department of Medicine, Duke University Health System, Durham, North Carolina

JENNIFER K. PHILLIPS, MD
Associate Chair and Associate Professor, Department of Family and Community Medicine, The University of New Mexico, Albuquerque, New Mexico

BETH POTTER, MD
Associate Professor, Department of Family Medicine and Community Health, University of Wisconsin-Madison School of Medicine and Public Health, University of Wisconsin-Madison, Madison, Wisconsin

JEFFREY D. QUINLAN, MD, FAAFP
Associate Professor, Chair, Department of Family Medicine, F. Edward Hebert School of Medicine, Uniformed Services University of the Health Sciences, Bethesda, Maryland

KRISTEN RUNDELL, MD, FAAFP
Vice Chair of Education, Associate Professor, Department of Family Medicine, The Ohio State University, Columbus, Ohio

KRISTEN RUSSELL, MSW, LCSW
Outpatient Clinical Social Work, Department of Case Management, Duke Child and Adolescent Gender Care, Duke University Health System, Durham, North Carolina

SARINA SCHRAGER, MD, MS
Professor, Department of Family Medicine and Community Health, University of Wisconsin-Madison School of Medicine and Public Health, University of Wisconsin-Madison, Madison, Wisconsin

JESSICA SERVEY, MD
Associate Professor, Department of Family Medicine, Associate Dean, Faculty Development, F. Edward Hebert School of Medicine, Uniformed Services University of the Health Sciences, Bethesda, Maryland

JESSICA R. STUMBO, MD, CAQSM
Primary Care Sports Medicine Fellowship, KentuckyOne Health, Associate Professor, Department of Family and Geriatric Medicine, Centers for Primary Care, University of Louisville, Louisville, Kentucky

EMILY TORELL, MD
Academic Fellow, Department of Family Medicine and Community Health,
University of Wisconsin-Madison School of Medicine and Public Health, University
of Wisconsin-Madison, Madison, Wisconsin

BELINDA A. VAIL, MD, MS, FAAFP
Professor and Chair, Department of Family Medicine, University of Kansas School of
Medicine, Kansas City, Kansas

CARISSA VAN DEN BERK CLARK, PhD, MSW
Assistant Professor, Department of Family and Community Medicine, School of Medicine,
Saint Louis University, St Louis, Missouri

Contents

Women's reproductive health maintenance begins in the early years of growth and development. Routine care is the basis for early detection of menstrual dysfunction and delays or acceleration of physical development. Patients and their families may not address menstruation concerns because of the sensitive nature of the topic, the patient's self-conscious attitudes, and the parent's apprehension. Providers should be able to provide early detection of menstrual abnormalities, which may uncover underlying health concerns and structural abnormalities. Early intervention and treatment may accelerate or decelerate physical growth, preserve fertility, and promote healthy behaviors with decreased psychological stress for patients and families.

Patients commonly present with unintended pregnancy in the primary care setting, and 1 in 4 women has an abortion in her lifetime. Early abortion services can be safely provided in the primary care setting. Abortion options provided in primary care settings include both medication abortion and early uterine aspiration abortion. Medication abortion, provided up to 10 weeks' gestational age, includes mifepristone (a progestin antagonist) and misoprostol (a prostaglandin). Uterine aspiration can be provided via manual or electronic vacuum in the first trimester.

The female athlete triad is a condition seen in physically active female athletes, consisting of low energy availability, menstrual dysfunction, and low bone mineral density. The condition should be viewed as a metabolic injury. It can have an impact on female athletes at any age or level. Activities at highest risk are those emphasizing leanness, aesthetics, and endurance. The cornerstone of treatment is improving mismatched energy balance. A multidisciplinary team, including health care providers, dieticians, and mental health professionals, is vital in caring for female athlete triad patients. Increased awareness and education are needed for medical as well as athletic communities.

Best Practices in Transgender Health: A Clinician's Guide

Jessica Lapinski, Tiffany Covas, Jennifer M. Perkins, Kristen Russell,
Deanna Adkins, Melanie Camejo Coffigny, and Sharon Hull

> Providing culturally competent and medically knowledgeable care to the
> transgender community is increasingly falling within the realms of practice
> for primary care providers. The purpose of this article is to provide an over-
> view of best practices as they relate to transgender care. This article is by
> no means a comprehensive guide, but rather a starting point for clinicians
> as they provide high-quality care to their transgender patients.

Plastic Surgery for Women

Michelle M. De Souza, Andrea D. Jewell, Samuel N. Grief, and Belinda A. Vail

> Plastic surgery is a broad field, including maxillofacial surgery, reconstruc-
> tion after injuries, hand surgery, and skin flaps and grafts, but the most
> common procedures for women are liposuction and body contouring,
> breast surgery, and facial cosmetic procedures. Techniques of face and
> brow lifts, blepharoplasty, and rhinoplasty are discussed as well as botu-
> linum toxin and filler injections, and laser and pulsed light techniques that
> may delay or eliminate the need for surgery. Comparison of the surgeries
> for breast reconstruction, reduction, augmentation, and mastopexy is
> discussed. New surgeries for enhancement of female genitalia are also
> examined.

Integrative Health for Women

Jennifer K. Phillips, Stephanie A. Cockrell, and Alisha N. Parada

> Integrative Medicine is a model of health care that combines both conven-
> tional and unconventional therapies that serve the whole person and focus
> on prevention and whole health. Women are the highest utilizers of health
> care and Integrative Medicine for a variety of reasons. Integrative Medicine
> represents a more "female energy" in the field of medicine, which is
> needed even more today as health care moves toward value-based care
> and out of high-cost and high-harm care. Integrative Medicine can be
> incorporated into medical practice and into health workers' lives for
> wellness.

**Medication-Assisted Treatment Considerations for Women with Opiate Addiction
Disorders**

Alicia A. Jacobs and Michelle Cangiano

> Opioid addiction rates are at a national high, with significant morbidity and
> mortality. In women, rates have been steadily increasing to be at par with
> addiction rates in men. Women tend to have quicker addiction and shorter
> duration to adverse outcomes. Treatment of women has the best out-
> comes when it is gender-specific, trauma-informed, connected with ac-
> cess to psychiatric services, and integrated into the medical home.
> Improved outcomes can be achieved with coordinated systems of care
> based on the harm-reduction model, with integration of medication-
> assisted therapy in a patient-centered medical home.

Women's Health

PRIMARY CARE:
CLINICS IN OFFICE PRACTICE

SERIES OF RELATED INTEREST

Medical Clinics (http://www.medical.theclinics.com)
Physician Assistant Clinics (http://www.physicianassistant.theclinics.com)
Obstetrics and Gynecology Clinics (https://www.obgyn.theclinics.com/)

THE CLINICS ARE AVAILABLE ONLINE!
Access your subscription at:
www.theclinics.com

Foreword

Emerging Challenges and Opportunities in Women's Health

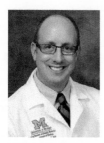

Joel J. Heidelbaugh, MD, FAAFP, FACG
Consulting Editor

The evolution of women's health as a subspecialty has brought substantial attention to the unique needs of women across the life cycle. This successful attention has spanned primary care and specialty care alike, yet more attention and education are needed in primary care realms to meet new challenges in women's health. As primary care services continue to expand, health care providers require resources and guidelines to deliver an excellent standard of care for women in the coming years.

In many ways, women are impressively more in tune with their health care needs when compared with men. They engage in more media presentations and publications about health, wellness, and nutrition than men. They attend more preventive health visits, engage with more cancer screening, and, on the whole, eat healthier than men and are more likely to embrace integrative health provisions. This issue of *Primary Care: Clinics in Office Practice* highlights the important topics of reproduction and issues surrounding providing termination services in the primary care setting. Primary care continues to be the central home for women to receive these services, and current education efforts are being directed at augmenting training in contraception and abortion procedures.

In 2018, practical knowledge lags behind in staying current in how to care for various populations of women across primary care settings. This issue contains articles that highlight the unique needs of female athletes, women in the military, and transgender patients. As the opioid crisis continues to mount, the need for caring for women with dependence issues is also escalating. Many patients who are diagnosed with cancer ultimately have the majority of their health care directed by their oncologists, yet primary care providers are still central to overall preventive and mental health care. New guidelines and medications for treating menopause and osteoporosis are presented. For women who undergo plastic surgery, either restorative or cosmetic,

Prim Care Clin Office Pract 45 (2018) xi–xii
https://doi.org/10.1016/j.pop.2018.10.002
0095-4543/18/© 2018 Published by Elsevier Inc.

primarycare.theclinics.com

various implications and complications are discussed as this importance is paramount given the rise of cosmetic surgeries performed outside of the United States.

I would like thank Drs Emily M. Godfrey and Diane M. Harper as well as the many dedicated authors for their valiant efforts in creating a very unique issue of articles for this issue of the *Primary Care: Clinics in Office Practice*. This information is timely and practical and can greatly augment the care of women across the life cycle and unique circumstances who we see in our daily practices.

Joel J. Heidelbaugh, MD, FAAFP, FACG
Departments of Family Medicine and Urology
University of Michigan Medical School
Ann Arbor, MI 48103, USA

Ypsilanti Health Center
200 Arnet, Suite 200
Ypsilanti, MI 48198, USA

E-mail address:
jheidel@umich.edu

Preface

Optimizing Women's Health in Primary Care

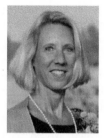
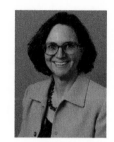

Diane M. Harper, MD, MPH, MS   Emily M. Godfrey, MD, MPH
Editors

Primary care providers are at the front lines of health care in the United States. They are in a position to address the first appearing risk factors whose treatment will prevent subsequent lethal diseases. In addition, primary care providers are frequently the safety net for marginalized populations who otherwise lack access to adequate care. As medical technology advances and lives are extended, primary care physicians continue to be the backbone of timely and preventive care services to diverse populations.

Adolescent and adult women account for more than 40% of visits annually to primary care offices. Their unique health care needs are often at odds with current legal rulings of political positioning. Regardless, human beings require humane access to health care, which is most often with the primary care provider. This encumbers an additional ethical duty for continuing education in implementation of new health knowledge for all persons.

The Women's Health issue of *Primary Care: Clinics in Office Practice* focuses on common health issues for which concise information for primary care is not readily available. We have included evidence-based guidance for diverse populations and conditions, including female athletes, cancer survivors, military women, transgender persons, and those presenting for management of reproductive life cycle transitions, unplanned pregnancy, opiate addiction, and integrative health. Each article was written to assist primary care providers to optimally manage women of every reproductive life stage.

Prim Care Clin Office Pract 45 (2018) xiii–xiv
https://doi.org/10.1016/j.pop.2018.10.001
0095-4543/18/© 2018 Published by Elsevier Inc.

primarycare.theclinics.com

This issue would not have been possible without the dedication and expertise of our authors. We wish to thank wholeheartedly each author for their enduring commitment to this work.

Diane M. Harper, MD, MPH, MS
Department of Family Medicine
Obstetrics and Gynecology
University of Michigan
1018 Fuller Street
Ann Arbor, MI 48104, USA

Emily M. Godfrey, MD, MPH
Family Medicine
Obstetrics and Gynecology
University of Washington
4311 11th Avenue Northeast, Suite 210
Box 354982
Seattle, WA 98105, USA

E-mail addresses:
diane.m.harper@gmail.com (D.M. Harper)
godfreye@uw.edu (E.M. Godfrey)

Being Reproductive

Kristen Rundell, MD*, Bethany Panchal, MD

KEYWORDS

- Puberty • Amenorrhea • Abnormal uterine bleeding • Polycystic ovarian syndrome

KEY POINTS

- Check growth, calculate expected adult height, record tanner stage and menstrual history at each visit.
- Initiate work-up for precocious puberty prior to age 8.
- Initiate work-up for primary amenorrhea if greater than 15 years of age without menstrual cycle.
- Treat polycystic ovarian disease with weight loss and oral contraceptives.

BECOMING REPRODUCTIVE

Women's reproductive health maintenance begins in the early years of growth and development with thorough monitoring by clinicians with an astute understanding of normal physiology and development. Routine continuity of care is the basis for early detection of menstrual dysfunction and delays or acceleration of physical development. Patients and their families may not address menstruation concerns due to the sensitive nature of the topic caused by the patient's self-conscious attitudes and/or parent's apprehension. A caring and competent provider will be able to provide early detection of menstrual abnormalities, which may uncover underlying health concerns and structural abnormalities. The early intervention and treatment may accelerate or decelerate physical growth, preserve fertility, and promote healthy behaviors with decreased psychological stress for the patient and her family.

PUBERTY AND FUNCTIONAL MENSTRUATION

Functional menstruation parameters have changed minimally over the years. The mean age of menarche, initiation of menstruation, is 12 to 13 years of age for well-nourished adolescent girls in developed countries. This is 2 years after thelarche or the development of breast tissue. (Tanner stage IV).[1–5] Some mild variations in onset of these changes is seen with different populations. For example, non-Hispanic black

Disclosure: The authors have nothing to disclose.
Department of Family Medicine, The Ohio State University, 2231 North High Street, Columbus, OH 43201, USA
* Corresponding author.
E-mail address: Kristen.Rundell@osumc.edu

adolescents achieve menarche 5.5 months earlier than adolescent girls of other races or ethnicities.[6] Socioeconomic conditions, psychological stressors, physical activity, medications, and underlying medical conditions may also influence the onset of menarche.[7] Increasing body mass index (BMI) has also led to an acceleration of pubertal development.[8,9]

The functional menstruation cycle is based on an intact hypothalamic-pituitary-ovarian axis. This axis is sensitive to physiologic, pathologic, and psychological changes.[10] The initiation of the cycle is by hypothalamus via pulsatile release of gonadotropin-releasing hormone (GnRH) to the pituitary, which produces follicle-stimulating hormone (FSH) and luteinizing hormone (LH). FSH works directly on ovarian follicles to produce estrogen. Estrogen stimulates the endometrium to proliferate, and LH prompts ovulation.

Once this cycle has been initiated, the beginning of menses should occur within 2 years. The average cycle is usually 21 to 45 days in length.[11] The average blood loss is 30 mL (2 tablespoons) per cycle and greater than 80 mL (one-third cup) is concerning for resulting anemia. Although it can be difficult for an adolescent to properly quantify her blood loss, comparing the amount of blood loss to typical units of measure such as tablespoons or cups can be helpful. Typical pad or tampon use should be 3 to 6 per day. If the patient is changing pads or tampons every 1 to 2 hours because of saturation, this is considered excessive and requires further evaluation.[12,13]

ABNORMAL PUBERTY AND DYSFUNCTIONAL MENSTRUATION

To accurately detect disorders in puberty and menstruation, a complete history including family history such as age of maternal menarche, social history, and physical examination should be done annually. Tanner staging, established in 1962, is still used to document physical and secondary sexual characteristic development. The American College of Obstetrics and Gynecology (ACOG) suggests that menses should be considered a routine vital sign for well child examinations starting at age 7 to 8 and continue as part of the well examination annually.[13] This helps set the expectations for patients and their families for normal development and screens for abnormalities in a confidential and open environment.[14] Once menses has occurred, the length of each cycle, days of menstruation, and heaviness of flow should be evaluated annually. Tracking height is also important in the continued evaluation of normal development. The equation for expected adult height is mother's height + father's height − 13 cm/2.[15,16] For children younger than 2 years old, the recommendation is to use the World Health Organization (WHO) growth charts. For children older than 2 years, the US Centers for Disease Control and Prevention (CDC) growth charts are the standard. Normal growth velocity should be 5 cm/y from age 4 to puberty, with peak height velocity of 8.3 cm/y 2 years prior to menarche. It is expected that girls will grow an average of 7 cm after menarche.[2–4,7,11,14,17,18] For children who are below the third percentile on the growth chart, the clinician should evaluate for malnutrition and systemic illness. For children who consistently exceed 97th percentile on the growth chart, an endocrine disorder may be suspected. Delay in growth is usually brought to the attention of a provider early; excess growth or tallness is usually not noted as an abnormality, and delays in determining pathology may exist.

PRECOCIOUS PUBERTY

Precocious puberty is defined by development of secondary sexual characteristics in girls younger than 8 years.[19,20] Up to 20% of black and 10% of white girls may have breast bud development by age 7 to 8.[21–25] More than 50% of early physical development cases are idiopathic, and the child will progress to menarche normally. Of the 5% to 10% who will have central precocious puberty, these may be caused by congenital anomalies, infection, neoplasm, or trauma to the central nervous system.[26] The major concern with advanced development is that the growth plates will close prematurely, and the maximum height will not be achieved.[19,26] Factors that may influence precocious puberty include race, age of maternal menarche, low birth weight, or early childhood obesity.[27,28] **Box 1** lists the initial work up of precocious puberty.

Once menstruation begins, the growth plates begin to close. For patients who experience precocious puberty, this may lead to premature closure of the growth plates and provide a short window for intervention. GnRH analogues (eg, leuprolide) appear to safely prevent premature fusion of growth plates. The risks, benefits, and costs of treatment need to be carefully reviewed with patients and their families **(Table 1)**.[30,31]

DELAYED PUBERTY

As distressing as precocious puberty is to patients, a diagnosis of delayed puberty has its own psychological and physical concerns. The clinical definition of delay of puberty is the absence of breast development by age 13 and lack of menses by age 15. The work up is similar for precocious puberty with the addition of prolactin and insulin-like growth factor I **(Box 2)**.[33,34]

The diagnosis of constitutional delay is made with LH or FSH in the prepubertal range (LH 5–25 IU/L, FSH 0–4.0 IU/L)[35] and assumes that the patient does not have a history of radiation, trauma or brain neoplasm, chronic disease, or a consistent documented delay of bone age. Only the girls with constitutional delay of growth and puberty or GnRH deficiency should be considered for therapy with overnight transdermal estradiol for 3 to 6 months **(Table 2)**. If spontaneous puberty or pubertal progress has not occurred in 4 to 6 months, a referral to pediatric endocrinologist is suggested.[33] The percentage of girls with short stature due to abnormal puberty is equal to the percentage of those with tall stature.

Most girls with tall stature do not seek medical intervention. High-dose sex steroid therapy has been used to promote growth plate closure in the past but has been decreasing in use because of adverse effects.[37] Adverse effects from high-dose estrogen include weight gain, nausea, increased vaginal discharge, benign breast changes,

---

Box 1
Initial work up for precocious puberty

Complete history including prenatal history

Family history, including maternal age of menarche

Medications (over the counter and herbals), chemotherapy, neuroleptics

Social history including history of head trauma

Serum levels of LH, FSH, estradiol, and thyroid-stimulating hormone (TSH) monitored every 6 months

Dehydroepiandrosterone sulfate (DHEAS) and 17-hydroxyprogesterone if hyperandrogenic

Radiographic imaging of growth plates

Head MRI if headache, vision changes, or seizures

Data from Refs.[20,27,29]

Table 1 Treatment for precocious puberty		
	Adverse Effects	**Cost[a]**
GnRH analogues (eg, leuprolide) 50 mcg/kg/d subcutaneously, increase by 10 mcg/kg/d each week until downregulation	Bone density loss, hot flashes, headaches, emotional lability	$846.00

[a] Cost may vary according to medical coverage.
Data from Refs.[30–32]

thrombosis, and possible decreased fertility because of primary ovarian insufficiency.[34] If the underlying cause is gigantism, then the treatment with octreotide and pegvisomant may be used to suppress growth hormone (GH).[38] Octreotide suppresses LH's response to GnRH and reduces GH and/or IGF-I (somatomedin C) in acromegaly. Pegvisomant selectively binds to the growth hormone (GH) receptors and causes a decrease in serum concentrations of IGF-I.[39]

ABNORMAL UTERINE BLEEDING IN THE ADOLESCENT

Abnormal uterine bleeding (AUB) is common in the adolescent patient, as it may take up to 24 months after the onset of menarche for regular ovulatory cycles to occur. As the differential diagnosis is extensive, a systematic approach is used for the diagnosis known by the acronym PALM–COEIN: polyp, adenomyosis, leiomyoma, malignancy and hyperplasia, coagulopathy, ovulatory dysfunction, endometrial, iatrogenic, and not yet classified. PALM–COEIN was introduced in 2011 by the International Federation of Gynecology and Obstetrics (FIGO).[40] PALM diagnoses relate to structural causes of AUB, whereas COEIN relates to non-structural causes. The work-up for AUB is listed in **Box 3**. The common terminologies used for the menstrual irregularities are defined in **Table 3**. The term dysfunctional uterine bleeding or DUB is no longer used and has been replaced by abnormal uterine bleeding for consistency.[41]

Box 2
Initial work up for delayed puberty

Complete history including prenatal history

Family history, including maternal age of menarche

Medications (over the counter and herbals), chemotherapy, neuroleptics

Social history including history of head trauma

Serum levels LH, FSH, estradiol, and TSH monitored every 6 months

Dehydroepiandrosterone sulfate (DHEAS) and 17-hydroxyprogesterone if hyperandrogenic

Radiographic imaging of growth plates

Head MRI if neurologic symptoms of headache, vision changes, or seizures.

Prolactin level

Insulin growth factor I

Data from Kaplowitz PB. Delayed puberty. Pediatr Rev 2010;31(5):189–95; and de Waal WJ, Greyn-Fokker MH, Stijnen T, et al. Accuracy of final height prediction and effect of growth-reductive therapy in 362 constitutionally tall children. J Clin Endocrinol Metab 1996;81(3):1206–16.

Table 2		
Treatment for delayed puberty caused by constitutional delay of growth and puberty		
	Side Effects	Cost[a]
Estradiol transdermal 6.2 mcg overnight for 3–6 mo	Edema, weight gain, headache, site irritation	$89/month

[a] Cost may vary according to medical coverage.
Data from Refs.[31,33,36]

The key menstrual history questions that a clinician should ask to establish AUB are related to determining whether the bleeding disorder is anovulatory or ovulatory. Anovulatory bleeding is characterized by periods that occur at irregular intervals, and the flow may be light to very heavy. Anovulation is the most common cause of AUB in adolescents. Ovulatory bleeding is characterized by periods that occur at regular intervals (every 21–35 days), but the flow is excessive, or the duration is greater than 7 days. This may signify a uterine polyp or thyroid or bleeding disorder. **Box 3** describes the initial work-up for AUB.

The concern for prolonged anovulatory cycles is the increased risk of endometrial cancer or hyperplasia. Although infrequent, with 0.2 cases per 100,000 women under the age 20 years, endometrial carcinoma may be diagnosed in adolescent patients. Therefore, if patients have anovulatory cycles for 2 to 3 years, morbid obesity, and all medical treatments have failed after thorough investigation or other potential causes, an endometrial biopsy should be obtained.[41]

For patients with ovulatory-related bleeding, clinicians should include questions related to past medication use and history of easy bruising or excessive bleeding after procedures or family history of coagulopathies. The most common bleeding disorder in women is von Willebrand disease, and heavy menses may be the first symptom of the underlying concerns.

Treatment for AUB depends on the goals for therapy. Hormonal treatment is frequently the mainstay of treatment for adolescents with anovulatory bleeding, because it corrects the underlying hormone imbalance. Prescribed hormonal options include combination estrogen/progestin hormonal contraceptives, such as the pill, patch, or vaginal ring, and progestin-only treatments. Progestin-only treatments include: levonorgestrel-releasing intrauterine system (LNG-IUS), medroxyprogesterone acetate, megestrol acetate, norethindrone acetate (minipill), etonorgestrel

Box 3
Initial work-up for abnormal uterine bleeding

Complete history to determine ovulatory versus anovulatory bleeding

Family history, including history of bleeding disorders

Medications (over the counter and herbals)

Physical examination including BMI and evaluation for hirsutism

Social history, including history of sexual activity and sexually transmitted infections

Pregnancy test, TSH, prolactin, coagulopathy laboratory tests, if indicated

Data from Palmert MR, Dunkel L. Clinical practice. Delayed puberty. N Engl J Med 2012;366(5):443–53; and Sweet M, Schmidt-Dalton T, Weiss P, et al. Evaluation and management of abnormal uterine bleeding in premenopausal women. Am Fam Physician 2012;85(1):35–43.

Table 3 Common terminologies used for the menstrual irregularities	
Anovulatory Abnormal Uterine Bleeding	**Ovulatory Abnormal Uterine Bleeding**
Amenorrhea- absence of periods for more than three cycles Oligomenorrhea- menses occurring intervals of more than 35 d Metrorrhagia- menses at irregular intervals with excessive bleeding or >7 d	Menorrhagia- menses at regular intervals with excessive bleeding or >7 d

Data from Committee on Practice Bulletins—Gynecology. Practice bulletin no. 136: management of abnormal uterine bleeding associated with ovulatory dysfunction. Obstet Gynecol 2013;122(1):176–85.

subdermal implant (eg, Nexplanon) and depo-medroxy progestone acetate.[41] Combined hormonal methods are the easiest to use, assuming the patient has no contraindications according to the US Medical Eligibility Criteria for Contraceptive Use recommendations.[42] Progestin-only methods are more appropriate, especially when estrogen-containing medications are contraindicated for patients with certain medical conditions, such as presence of thrombogenic mutations, (ie, factor V Leiden mutation).[42]

For ovulatory bleeding, goals of treatment usually include reducing blood flow. This can be achieved with several treatments, including exogenous hormones, nonsteroidal anti-inflammatory (NSAID) medications, or antifibrinolyics, which are competitive inhibitors of plasminogen activation.[43] Treatment with estrogen-progestin contraceptives and LNG-IUS 52 mg are considered the first line of treatment, followed by high-dose oral or injectable progestin-only medications.[43] Treatment with antifibrinolyics, such as tranexamic acid, is often reserved for those who have failed other treatments first.[39] **Table 4** lists commonly used treatments for AUB for adolescents.

AMENORRHEA IN THE ADOLESCENT

Amenorrhea in the adolescent has a broad differential, and this article will focus on primary amenorrhea or the failure to reach menarche. Primary amenorrhea includes adolescents without breast development by age 13, no menses by age 15, or no menses at age 14 with signs of hirsutism. The work-up for primary and secondary amenorrhea is essentially the same (**Box 4**). Primary amenorrhea is commonly caused by genetic or chromosomal abnormalities, leading to primary ovarian insufficiency.

The treatment goal is to initiate the start of puberty if possible, for the continued normal development of the adolescent. It is also important to minimize the consequences of the hypoestrogenic state and maintain future fertility. Lack of estrogen may result in decreased height and bone development, which can be alleviated by replacement estrogen formulations, such as combined hormonal contraception. The treatment of primary amenorrhea is based on the underlying pathology, whether it is hormonal, nutritional, or functional.

Polycystic Ovarian Syndrome in Adolescents

Polycystic ovarian syndrome (PCOS) is the most common cause of anovulatory AUB in adolescents. It has also been linked to infertility and has lifelong metabolic and endocrinologic implications.[44] It has been estimated to affect 5% to 10% of women of reproductive age. The criterion for diagnosis in adolescents was established in 2015 by several international pediatric subspecialty societies.[45] **Box 5** summarizes

Being Reproductive   593

Table 4 Treatment for abnormal uterine bleeding		
	Side Effects	Cost[a]
Combined hormonal contraception (includes pills, transdermal patch, or vaginal ring)	Weight changes, nausea, headaches	$14.00/mo
Progestin-only pills: Medroxyprogesterone acetate 5–10 mg/d for 12–14 d or 5 mg/d continuously Norethindrone 5–15 mg/d for 21 d	Dizziness, headache, breast tenderness	$36.00/mo
Levonorgestrel-releasing intrauterine system 52 mg	Irregular bleeding, bloating, breast tenderness	$562.00 $50.00 340b price
Etononorgestrel subdermal implant (Nexplanon)	Irregular bleeding, headache, depressed mood	Up to $1300
Nonsteroidal anti-inflammatory drugs: Mefenamic acid 500 mg twice daily for 4–5 d Naproxen 250–500 mg twice daily for 4–5 d Ibuprofen 600–1200 mg daily for 4–5 d	Nausea, vomiting, gastrointestinal hemorrhage	$14.00
Tranexamic acid 1300 mg orally 3 times daily during menses for up to 5 d	Headaches, MSK pain, nausea	$149.99 for 30–650 mg tablets

[a] Cost may vary according to medical coverage.
Data from Refs.[28,32,43]

these criteria. Evaluation for PCOS should be considered in any adolescent girl with the following signs or symptoms: hirsutism, treatment-resistant acne, menstrual irregularities (see **Box 1** for AUB), or morbid obesity. Girls diagnosed with PCOS should undergo annual screening for insulin resistance, dyslipidemia, and obesity.

The treatment of PCOS is based on the individual patient's treatment goals. Treatment is usually focused on correcting menstrual irregularities, cutaneous manifestations of hyperandrogenism, and/or addressing the metabolic comorbidities associated with PCOS. First-line treatment involves the use of combined estrogen/progestin hormonal contraceptives to regulate endometrial cycling, thus protecting against endometrial carcinoma and inhibition of ovarian function and normalizing androgen excess.[44] Clinicians should address comorbidities by focusing on lifestyle modifications, such as weight loss and exercise. The addition of metformin as part

Box 4 Initial work-up for primary or secondary amenorrhea
Detailed history, including eating and exercising habits
Physical examination, including palpation of thyroid, BMI, evaluation of hirsutism,
Documentation of dysmorphic features
Pregnancy test, LH, FSH, TSH, free and total testosterone, DHEAS
Complete blood cell count (CBC) and chemistry panel
Pelvic ultrasound for anatomy, MRI for pituitary dysfunction, thyroid ultrasound
If no uterus present, referral for chromosomal testing is suggested
Data from Refs.[20,37,41]

Box 5
Diagnostic criteria of polycystic ovarian syndrome in adolescents

Otherwise unexplained combination of:

1. Abnormal uterine bleeding Pattern
   a. Abnormal for age or gynecologic age
   b. Persistence of symptoms for 1 to 2 years

2. Evidence of hyperandrogenism
   a. Persistent testosterone elevation above adult norms
   b. Moderate-severe hirsutism is clinical evidence of hyperandrogenism
   c. Moderate-severe inflammatory acne vulgaris may be hyperandrogenemia

Data from Rosenfield RL. The diagnosis of polycystic ovary syndrome in adolescents. Pediatrics 2015;136:1154–65.

---

of the treatment plan may be beneficial in some, particularly if glucose intolerance is evident.[46]

MENSTRUATION IN SPECIAL POPULATIONS
Patients with Physical and Developmental Delays

Up to 8.4% of adolescents have developmental and/or physical disabilities, which may be associated menstrual disorders in the adolescent. Patients with developmental and physical disabilities have more menstrual disorders related to anovulatory bleeding. This may be related to adverse effects of medications for mood and behavior, which can increase the prolactin level, causing oligomenorrhea. Patients taking valproic acid may be more likely to be diagnosed with PCOS.[47] Patients with autism spectrum conditions may experience a slight delay in the onset of menarche due to poor nutrition or delayed growth. For many patients and their families, the conversation regarding goals for menstrual regulation needs to include the desire for decreased or absent menstrual cycles, possible changes in mood and the need for long or short term contraception.[47,48] This discussion will determine the best medical option. Many adolescents with physical disabilities may have difficulty managing menstrual blood flow and hygiene. ACOG provides guidelines for menstrual suppression, if that is the desired outcome of the patient and family. Initially, NSAIDs may decrease menstrual bleeding by up to 40%. Continuous combined hormonal contraceptives will achieve menstrual suppression, yet it is not recommended for patients for whom estrogen is a contraindication.[42] Continuous use means that the patient takes only the active pills and skips the hormone-free week. Likewise, the vaginal ring can be used continuously without a hormone-free week. The contraceptive patch is not recommended for continuous use. Progestin-only pills are an option, yet should be taken at the same time daily to avoid breakthrough bleeding. Depot medroxyprogesterone acetate (DMPA), an injectable given every 3 months, often provides complete menstrual suppression after the second or third dose. However, weight gain is an unfortunate side effect with this medication. Levonorgestrel intrauterine system (LNG-IUS) is an alternative to daily oral medications. LNG-IUS may be more cost-effective and convenient for patients than treatments that require daily or quarterly administration. There are several US Food and Drug Administration (FDA)-approved LNG-IUS types available, the 52 mg, 19.5 mg and 13.5 mg-all containing levonorgestrel; providers should work with the patient to decide on which LNG-IUS is best for her. A progestin-only subdermal implant may be used; however, only about one-third of users actually experience amenorrhea, and another third may have irregular bleeding.[49] **Table 5** summarizes these options with the associated

Table 5
Treatment for menstrual suppression

	Concerns	Cost/mo
Antiprostaglandin (NSAID) medications	Not complete suppression	<$5.00
Continuous combined hormonal contraceptives (pills or ring)	Need to take continuously	$14.00
Progestin-only pills	Breakthrough bleeding	$36.00
DMPA	Weight gain	$50.00
LNG-IUS	Insertion procedure, office procedure	$50-$562.00 (one time)
Subdermal implants	Breakthrough bleeding, office procedure	

Costs may vary depending on location and insurance. All medication information including costs was obtained from Committee on Practice Bulletins—Gynecology. Practice bulletin no. 136: management of abnormal uterine bleeding associated with ovulatory dysfunction. Obstet Gynecol 2013;122(1):176–85 compiled from www.epocrates.com, Micromedex, and www.goodrx.com.
Data from Refs.[28,32,47,48,50]

patient concerns. Endometrial ablation and suppression prior to menarche are not considered treatment options. Hysterectomy for menstrual suppression is only to be considered if there are no other viable options.[47,48]

SUMMARY

Dysfunction in normal growth and development has physical, psychological, and reproductive implications for adolescent girls. Routine monitoring of growth and development parameters and open conversations with patients and their families will help detect early dysfunction and concerns so that early evaluations may be completed and interventions instituted.

REFERENCES

1. Chumlea WC, Schubert CM, Roche AF, et al. Age at menarche and racial comparisons in US girls. Pediatrics 2003;111:110–3.
2. Bordini B, Rosenfield RL. Normal pubertal development: part II: clinical aspects of puberty. Pediatr Rev 2011;32(7):281–92, 3.
3. Chulani VL, Gordon LP. Adolescent growth and development. Prim Care 2014; 41(3):465–87.
4. Holland-Hall C, Burstein GR. Adolescent development. In: Kliegman R, Stanton BF, St. Geme JW III, et al, editors. Nelson textbook of pediatrics. 20th edition. Philadelphia: Elsevier; 2016. p. 926–36.
5. Bordini B, Rosenfielf RL. Aspects of puberty. Pediatr Rev 2011;32(7):281–92, 3.
6. Apter D, Hermanson E. Update on female pubertal development. Curr Opin Obstet Gynecol 2002;14:475–81.
7. Biro FM, Huang B, Crawford PB, et al. Pubertal correlates in black and white girls. J Pediatr 2006;148(2):234–40.
8. Hickey M, Balen A. Menstrual disorders in adolescence: investigation and management. Hum Reprod Update 2003;9(5):493–504.

9. World Health Organization multicenter study on menstrual and ovulatory patterns in adolescent girls. I. A multicenter cross-sectional study of menarche. World Health Organization Task Force on Adolescent Reproductive Health. J Adolesc Health Care 1986;7:229–35.

10. Flug D, Largo RH, Prader A. Menstrual patterns in adolescent Swiss girls: a longitudinal study. Ann Hum Biol 1984;11:495–508.

11. Widholm O, Kantero RL. A statistical analysis of the menstrual patterns of 8,000 Finnish girls and their mothers. Acta Obstet Gynecol Scand Suppl 1971; 14(Suppl):1–36.

12. Chimbira TH, Anderson ABM. Relation between measured menstrual blood loss and patient's subjective assessment of loss, duration of bleeding, number of sanitary towels used, uterine weight and endometrial surface area. Br J Obstet Gynaecol 1980;87:603–9.

13. Committee Opinion No. 651. Menstruation in girls and adolescents: using the menstrual cycle as a vital sign. Obstet Gynecol 2015;126(6):1328.

14. Rogol AD, Hayden GF. Etiologies and early diagnosis of short stature and growth failure in children and adolescents. J Pediatr 2014;164(5 suppl):S1–14.e6.

15. Barstow C, Rerucha C. Evaluation of short and tall stature in children. Am Fam Physician 2015;92(1):43–50.

16. Bordini B, Rosenfield RL. Normal pubertal development: part I: the endocrine basis of puberty. Pediatr Rev 2011;32(6):223–9.

17. Tanner JM, Davies PS. Clinical longitudinal standards for height and height velocity for North American children. J Pediatr 1985;107(3):317–29.

18. Kaplowitz PB, Oberfield SE. Reexamination of the age limit for defining when puberty is precocious in girls in the United States: implications for evaluation and treatment. Drug and Therapeutics and Executive Committees of the Lawson Wilkins Pediatric Endocrine Society. Pediatrics 1999;104:936–41.

19. Styne DM, Grumbach MM. Physiology and disorders of puberty. In: Melmed S, Polonsky KS, Larsen PR, et al, editors. Williams textbook of endocrinology. 13th edition. Philadelphia: Elsevier; 2016. p. 1074–218.

20. Kaplowitz P, Bloch C, Section on Endocrinology, American Academy of Pediatrics. Evaluation and referral of children with signs of early puberty. Pediatrics 2016;137(1):1–6.

21. Herman-Giddens ME, Slora EJ, Wasserman RC, et al. Secondary sexual characteristics and menses in young girls seen in office practice: a study from the Pediatric Research in Office Settings network. Pediatrics 1997;99(4):505–12.

22. Wu T, Mendola P, Buck GM. Ethnic differences in the presence of secondary sex characteristics and menarche among US girls: the Third National Health and Nutrition Examination Survey, 1988–1994. Pediatrics 2002;110(4):752–7.

23. Rosenfield RL, Lipton RB, Drum ML. Thelarche, pubarche, and menarche attainment in children with normal and elevated body mass index [published correction appears in Pediatrics. 2009;123(4):1255]. Pediatrics 2009;123(1):84–8.

24. Biro FM, Galvez MP, Greenspan LC, et al. Pubertal assessment method and baseline characteristics in a mixed longitudinal study of girls. Pediatrics 2010; 126(3):e583–90.

25. De Leonibus C, Marcovecchio ML, Chiavaroli V, et al. Timing of puberty and physical growth in obese children: a longitudinal study in boys and girls. Pediatr Obes 2014;9(4):292–9.

26. Root AW. Precocious puberty. Pediatr Rev 2000;21(1):10–9.

27. Carel JC, Léger J. Clinical practice. Precocious puberty. N Engl J Med 2008; 358(22):2366–77.

28. Klein DA, Emerick JE, Sylvester JE, et al. Disorders in puberty: an approach to diagnosis and management. Am Fam Physician 2017;96(9):590–9.

29. Guaraldi F, Beccuti G, Gori D, et al. Management of endocrine disease: long-term outcomes of the treatment of central precocious puberty. Eur J Endocrinol 2016; 174(3):R79–87.

30. Carel JC, Eugster EA, Rogol A, et al, ESPE-LWPES GnRH Analogs Consensus Conference Group. Consensus statement on the use of gonadotropin-releasing hormone analogs in children. Pediatrics 2009;123(4):e752–62.

31. Palmert MR, Dunkel L. Clinical practice. Delayed puberty. N Engl J Med 2012; 366(5):443–53.

32. Sweet M, Schmidt-Dalton T, Weiss P, et al. Evaluation and management of abnormal uterine bleeding in premenopausal women. Am Fam Physician 2012; 85(1):35–43.

33. Kaplowitz PB. Delayed puberty. Pediatr Rev 2010;31(5):189–95.

34. de Waal WJ, Greyn-Fokker MH, Stijnen T, et al. Accuracy of final height prediction and effect of growth-reductive therapy in 362 constitutionally tall children. J Clin Endocrinol Metab 1996;81(3):1206–16.

35. Lab references from Available at: www.medlineplus.gov.

36. Menstrual manipulation for adolescents with physical and developmental disabilities. Obstet Gynecol 2016;128(2):e20–5.

37. Davies JH, Cheetham T. Investigation and management of tall stature. Arch Dis Child 2014;99(8):772–7.

38. Speroff L, Fritz MA. Clinical gynecologic endocrinology and infertility. 7th edition. Philadelphia: Lippincott Williams & Wilkins; 2005. 402, 547, 549, 553–6, 560–1, 566, 569, 628–9, 808, 811.

39. MicromedexÂ (electronic version). Greenwood Village (CO): Truven Health Analytics. Available at: http://www.micromedexsolutions.com/. Accessed April 15, 2018.

40. Munro MG, Critchley HO, Broder MS, et al. FIGO classification system (PALM-COEIN) for causes of abnormal uterine bleeding in nongravid women of reproductive age. FIGO Working Group on Menstrual Disorders. Int J Gynaecol Obstet 2011;113:3–13.

41. Committee on Practice Bulletins—Gynecology. Practice bulletin no. 136: management of abnormal uterine bleeding associated with ovulatory dysfunction. Obstet Gynecol 2013;122(1):176–85.

42. Curtis KM, Tepper NK, Jatlaoui TC, et al. U.S. medical eligibility criteria for contraceptive use, 2016. MMWR Recomm Rep 2016;65(3):1–104.

43. Matthews ML. Abnormal uterine bleeding in reproductive-aged women. Obstet Gynecol Clin North Am 2015;42(1):103–15.

44. Rosenfield RL. The diagnosis of polycystic ovary syndrome in adolescents. Pediatrics 2015;136:1154–65.

45. Agapova SE, Cameo T, Sopher AB, et al. Diagnosis and challenges of polycystic ovary syndrome in adolescence. Semin Reprod Med 2014;32(3):194–201.

46. Hoeger K, Davidson K, Kochman L, et al. The impact of metformin, oral contraceptives, and lifestyle modification on polycystic ovary syndrome in obese adolescent women in two randomized, placebo-controlled clinical trials. J Clin Endocrinol Metab 2008;93(11):4299–306.

47. Quint E. Menstrual and reproductive issues in adolescent with physical and developmental disabilities. Obstet Gynecol 2014;124(2 pt 1):367–75.

48. Bradley LD, Gueye NA. The medical management of abnormal uterine bleeding in reproductive aged women. Am J Obstet Gynecol 2016;214(1):31–44.

49. Zigler RE, McNicholas C. Unscheduled vaginal bleeding with progestin-only contraceptive use [review]. Am J Obstet Gynecol 2017;216(5):443–50.
50. Snyder AH, Weisman CS, Liu G, et al. The impact of the affordable care act on contraceptive use and costs among privately insured women. Womens Health Issues 2018;28(3):219–23.

Providing Abortion Services in the Primary Care Setting

Jennifer R. Amico, MD, MPH[a],*, Terri L. Cheng, MD[b], Emily M. Godfrey, MD, MPH[c,d]

KEYWORDS

- Abortion • Primary care • Unintended pregnancy • Family planning • Procedure

KEY POINTS

- Patients commonly present with unintended pregnancy in the primary care setting, and 1 in 4 women has an abortion in her lifetime.
- Early abortion services can be safely provided in the primary care setting.
- Abortion options provided in primary care settings include both medication abortion and early uterine aspiration abortion.
- Medication abortion, provided up to 10 weeks' gestational age, includes mifepristone (a progestin antagonist) and misoprostol (a prostaglandin).
- Uterine aspiration can be provided via manual or electronic vacuum in the first trimester.

INTRODUCTION

Most patients who seek primary care services make decisions about childbearing over the course of their lifetime, including planning or preventing pregnancy, so that they can control their desired number and spacing of children. Primary care clinicians see many women of reproductive age (15–44 years), who make up approximately 50 million preventive care visits per year.[1] The American Academy of Family Physicians (AAFP), American College of Obstetricians and Gynecologists, and the Disease Control and Prevention (CDC) recommend that primary care clinicians incorporate reproductive life planning for women of reproductive age.[2–4] Additionally, the CDC recently published recommendations about the delivery of quality family planning services in primary care settings.[5]

Disclosure: The authors have nothing to disclose.
[a] Department of Family Medicine and Community Health, Rutgers Robert Wood Johnson Medical School, 125 Paterson Street, MEB 262, New Brunswick, NJ 08901, USA; [b] Department of Family Medicine and Public Health, University of California San Diego, 200 West Arbor Drive #8201A, San Diego, CA 92103, USA; [c] Family Medicine, University of Washington, 4311 11th Avenue Northeast, Suite 210, Box 354982, Seattle, WA 98105, USA; [d] Obstetrics and Gynecology, University of Washington, 4311 11th Avenue Northeast, Suite 210, Box 354982, Seattle, WA 98105, USA
* Corresponding author.
E-mail address: jennifer.amico@rutgers.edu

Prim Care Clin Office Pract 45 (2018) 599–613
https://doi.org/10.1016/j.pop.2018.07.010
primarycare.theclinics.com

Approximately half of pregnancies in the United States are unintended.[6] Primary care providers who care for women of reproductive age should be able to manage patients with unintended pregnancy, including discussing a patient's reproductive life plan, determining the gestational age (GA) of the pregnancy, and a discussion of options (parenting, abortion, or adoption).

Abortion is common. Excluding miscarriages, approximately 40% of unintended pregnancies end in abortion,[6] numbering 1 million abortions provided in the United States per year.[7,8] One in 4 women has an abortion in her lifetime.[9] In 2014, the abortion rate among women ages 15 to 44 was the lowest rate since abortion was legalized in 1973.[7] Many women seeking abortion care are poor, with three-quarters low income and approximately half living below the federal poverty level.[10] Although white women make up the largest proportion of abortion patients (39%), black women and Hispanic women are both over-represented (28% and 25%, respectively).[10] A majority of abortion patients are in their 20s (60%), with minors making up fewer than 5% of those accessing abortion care.[10]

A vast majority of abortions occur early in pregnancy, with two-thirds occurring prior to 9 weeks' gestation and more than 90% during the first trimester.[11] In the primary care setting, early abortion can be provided by medication (up to 10 weeks) or by uterine aspiration (up to 12 weeks).[12–14] Abortion is exceedingly safe, with a major complication rate of less than 0.5%,[15] and risk of death of less than 1 in 100,000 procedures,[16] approximately 14 times less than the risk of death from a term pregnancy and delivery.[16] Despite the safety of abortion, the right to abortion in the United States is continuously challenged due to the current sociopolitical climate.

ABORTION POLICY AND RESTRICTIONS

The Supreme Court ruling in Roe v Wade in 1973 decided that women have the legal right to abortion in the United States until viability.[17] Subsequently, 2 additional rulings paved the way for states to pass legislative restrictions on abortion. The Hyde Amendment, passed by the House of Representatives in 1976 and upheld by the Supreme Court in 1980, barred the use of federal funds to pay for abortion.[18] Then in 1992, Planned Parenthood v Casey, which challenged the constitutionality of abortion restrictions in Pennsylvania, upheld Roe v Wade but ruled that states could regulate abortions as long as restrictions did not pose an "undue burden" on those seeking abortions.[19]

Currently, 90% of US counties have no abortion provider.[7] Since 2010, states have enacted 338 restrictions on abortion.[20] As of 2016, more than half of states have at least 4 of the 10 major types[a] of abortion restrictions, and 22 states have 6 or more major restrictions.[20] Clinicians who provide abortion care must be familiar with the specific regulations in their state.

In much of the world, abortion is illegal except under the strictest of circumstances.[21,22] In places where abortion is illegal, however, it is just as frequently performed but unsafe. As a result, unsafe abortions account for between 8% an 18% of maternal deaths worldwide and approximately 20,000 to 40,000 deaths yearly.[21,22] Compared with the United States, the risk of dying from abortion worldwide is 350 times higher and 800 times higher in sub-Saharan Africa.[22]

---

[a] Ten major abortion restrictions: parental involvement for minors; mandated counseling; waiting periods; mandated ultrasounds; bans on Medicaid funding; restricting abortion coverage in private health plans; medication abortion restrictions; regulations on abortion facilities; unconstitutional bans on abortion before viability; and enacting a preemptive ban on abortion if Roe v Wade is overturned.[20]

ABORTION PROVISION IN THE PRIMARY CARE SETTING

Both medication and uterine aspiration abortion fit within the scope of primary care.[13,14] Abortion care uses skills that primary care providers already have, such as patient-centered counseling, early pregnancy evaluation, miscarriage management techniques, paracervical block, and cervical dilation. In states that do not restrict their practice, advanced practice clinicians provide early abortion care as safely and effectively as physicians.[23,24] Medication abortion can be provided up to 10 weeks of pregnancy (70 days from last menstrual period [LMP]) and includes administration of mifepristone (a progestin antagonist, which stops the growth of the pregnancy) and misoprostol (a prostaglandin, which causes uterine cramping to expel the pregnancy).[25,26] First-trimester procedural abortion involves a uterine aspiration procedure, which can be performed with a manual vacuum aspirator or an electric vacuum aspirator.[14] Abortion patients report high satisfaction with abortion care within their primary care center, citing appreciation for the privacy, convenience, and continuity of care.[27,28]

Opportunities for abortion training within primary care residencies, in particular family medicine, has been increasing. The Society of Teachers of Family Medicine procedural training standards for family medicine residencies categorize uterine aspiration as a category A2 procedure, meaning that residents must have exposure during residency and the opportunity to train to competence, if desired.[29,30] Resident training in abortion leads to improved knowledge of early abortion, skills providing medication and uterine aspiration abortion, and increased intent to provide abortion care after graduation. Furthermore, residency training in abortion care also leads to improved early pregnancy ultrasound skills, contraceptive provision including intrauterine device (IUD) provision, and miscarriage management skills.[31–33]

COUNSELING AND COMMUNICATION ABOUT ABORTION

Pregnancy testing and counseling are considered a part of core family planning services, as outlined by the CDC quality family planning (QFP) guidelines.[5] The QFP guidelines detail standard of care for family planning services offered within the primary care setting and recommend that primary care providers know how to manage and counsel patients who present with unintended pregnancy.

Options counseling offers support and information needed to explore available alternatives to pregnancy and allows a patient to clarify values and emotions. It differs from abortion counseling, which is a discussion of the different methods of abortion, such as medication or aspiration abortion, and informed consent, which reviews the specific procedure, risks, anticipated benefits, and alternative therapeutic regimens.[34]

Abortion counseling has evolved as the field has faced significant challenges, primarily from the increasing stigmatization of abortion since legalization.[35] Several studies have demonstrated that a majority of patients seeking abortion report stigma in some form.[36,37] Clinicians providing options counseling and abortion counseling should be aware of the ways in which they may inadvertently perpetuate stigma and should use patient-centered language when talking about abortion and pregnancy decision making to maintain professionalism.

Pregnancy Options Counseling

Options counseling training for family medicine residents is recommended by the Accreditation Council for Graduate Medical Education and the AAFP and should be provided as recommended by the QFP guidelines (**Box 1**).[5,38] Primary care providers should discuss and give appropriate referrals for prenatal care, abortion, and adoption services.

> **Box 1**
> **Options counseling-starting points for discussion**
>
> How are you feeling about this pregnancy?
>
> Before you found out that you were pregnant, what were your feelings about abortion/adoption/parenting?
>
> Under what circumstances do you believe abortion/adoption/parenting is ok?
>
> Under what circumstances would you like to become a parent/have more children?
>
> What are your goals for the next year? How would each option help or hinder those goals?
>
> What is the worst thing you think could happen?
>
> How would you like things to turn out for you ideally?
>
> You've said what your partner's/parent's/community's beliefs are. Can you tell me more about what you believe?
>
> *Adapted from* Singer J. Options counseling: techniques for caring for women with unintended pregnancies. J Midwifery Womens Health. 2004;49(3):238, Baker A. Abortion and options counseling: A comprehensive reference. Granite City, IL: Hope Clinic for Women; 1995, National Abortion Federation. Unsure about your pregnancy? A guide to making the right decision for you [Internet]. *Available from*: https://www.prochoice.org/pubs_research/publications/downloads/are_you_pregnant/pregnancy_guide_english.pdf, and Runkle A. In good conscience: A practical, emotional, and spiritual guide to deciding whether to have an abortion. San Francisco, CA: Josey-Bass; 1998

Principles of options counseling should include

1. Active listening: the patient is responsible for self-exploration, assessing options, and ultimately making a decision. The role of the clinician is to listen actively, provide unbiased information, offer support, and assist in evaluating options while respecting the ethical principles of autonomy and self-determination.[34]
2. Providing accurate information: the clinician must have current and accurate information about available pregnancy options, including parenting, abortion, or adoption and any legal requirements.[39] Clinicians should ask patients what questions they have, try to determine patient perceptions and fears, and then address knowledge gaps in a manner that patients comprehend.[34]
3. Communication and counseling style: the provider should create a comfortable environment, be mindful of tone and body language, and use open-ended questions. Communication is enhanced by inviting a patient to express thoughts freely and validating the patient's emotions.[34]

Abortion Counseling

Abortion counseling includes offering abortion options either by medication or a uterine aspiration procedure. This should also include information about the pros and cons of each method, expected side effects, length of the abortion process, pain management, potential risks, resumption of normal activities, and follow-up care.[39,40]

Patients typically choose one abortion method over another based on personal preference. Some patients prefer the privacy and lesser invasiveness of a medication abortion, whereas others prefer the simplicity and shorter duration of discomfort of an aspiration abortion. Other details comparing the methods are listed in **Table 1**. Studies show greatest acceptability and satisfaction when patients are able to choose the type of abortion.[41]

Table 1
Early abortion options

	Medication Abortion	Uterine Aspiration Procedure
What are the advantages?	No injections, anesthesia, or instruments are needed.	Procedure can be completed in a few minutes and is effective 99% of the time.
	Patient may feel experience is more natural, similar to a miscarriage.	Patient encounters less bleeding compared with a medication abortion.
	Patient completes abortion at home, which may feel more private.	Medical staff members are available for support during the abortion.
	Patient can choose to be alone or have a support person.	Procedure can be done later in the pregnancy than a medication abortion.
What are the disadvantages?	It takes 1–2 d to complete the abortion.	A health care provider inserts instruments inside the uterus.
	Bleeding can be heavy and may last longer than with an aspiration abortion procedure.	Anesthetics and pain medicines may cause side effects.
	Cramps can be severe and may last longer than with an aspiration abortion.	Clinic policy may restrict who is allowed to accompany the patient in the procedure room.
	It cannot be done as late in pregnancy as an aspiration abortion.	The suction device may be noisy.
	It cannot end a tubal or ectopic pregnancy.	It cannot end a tubal or ectopic pregnancy.

From Reproductive Health Access Project. Early abortion options. Available at: https://www. reproductiveaccess.org/wp-content/uploads/2014/12/early_abortion_options.pdf. Accessed March 12, 2017; with permission.

Informed Consent for Abortion

Informed consent for abortion should review the risks, benefits, and alternatives to an abortion procedure as well as confirm that the abortion decision is voluntary.[40,42,43] Some special considerations for informed consent are discussed later.

State-required counseling

Many states have instituted waiting periods or counseling requirements prior to abortion procedures. This counseling may require the use of state-agency materials that can often contain erroneous and misleading information.[44–46] Although the stated objective of these requirements is to "ensure patients understand the risks of and alternatives to abortion," little evidence suggests they achieve those goals, enhance the quality of women's decision making, or improve postabortion well-being.[44,45] Primary care clinicians who choose to provide abortion care must familiarize themselves with abortion counseling requirements in their state.

Counseling minors

The American Academy of Pediatrics supports the right of adolescents to access confidential care when considering all pregnancy options.[47,48] Most minors ages 14 to 17 are able to competently provide consent to abortion and understand the risks and benefits of the options to make voluntary, rational, and independent decisions.[47,49,50] Nonetheless, most minors do involve a parent in their decision to end a pregnancy.[47] States differ on regulations about minors' rights to consent to abortion and other reproductive health services,[51] so clinicians should familiarize themselves with the specific regulations pertaining to their state.

PROVIDING ABORTION CARE
Clinical Evaluation Prior to Abortion

Pregnancy evaluation and gestational age determination

Medical assessment prior to abortion includes confirmation of the pregnancy and GA dating. GA assessment is needed to confirm appropriate limits for the available abortion methods.[39,40] GA can be accurately diagnosed with patient history of LMPs and use of clinical pelvic examination or ultrasound.[39,40] Although ultrasound is widely used, it is not required for first-trimester abortion.[52,53] Routine use of ultrasound has not been shown to improve the safety or efficacy of abortion but should be used when GA is uncertain or when there are symptoms of bleeding or pain.[53]

Medical history and testing

Routine medical history should be performed to identify contraindications or risk factors for complications related to the abortion procedure. Some medical conditions may not be appropriate for the primary care setting because of the need for monitoring in cases of severe cardiopulmonary disease or conditions that place patients at high risk of hemorrhage, such as placenta accreta or coagulopathy.[40,54] Other conditions, such as obesity or uterine fibroids, may require additional preprocedure planning but often are not contraindications for outpatient care.[40,55] Medical history should also include a risk assessment for violence or coercion.[39,40]

Contraindications to abortion

Contraindications to medication abortion are listed in **Box 2**. There are no absolute contraindications for aspiration of the uterus. Caution should be exercised, however, in patients who have uterine anomalies, coagulation problems, active pelvic infection, extreme anxiety, or any condition causing patients to be medically unstable.[40,54]

Laboratory testing

Most women presenting for abortion care in primary care settings do not require laboratory testing. Rh blood typing must be offered to administer Rh-immunoglobulin when indicated.[39] Hemoglobin or hematocrit should be offered, especially if a patient has history of anemia. Many providers offer sexually transmitted infection screening at the time of an abortion, but it is not required for provision of abortion.[5,43]

Box 2
Contraindications to medication abortion with mifepristone

Known or suspected ectopic pregnancy

Chronic adrenal failure or long-term corticosteroid therapy

Known hypersensitivity to medications

Hemorrhagic disorder or concurrent anticoagulant therapy

Inherited porphyria

IUD in place

Data from Danco Laboratories. Mifeprex prescribing information. Available at: https://www.earlyoptionpill.com/for-health-professionals/prescribing-mifeprex/prescribing-information/. Accessed March 12, 2017.

Methods of Abortion: Medication Abortion

The protocol for medication abortion with mifepristone and misoprostol was updated in March 2016 by the US Food and Drug Administration.[25] The new Food and Drug Administration protocol aligns with the evidence-based protocol for medication abortion, which includes the following regimen up to 70 days from LMP[25,26,56–58]:

- Day 1: mifepristone, 200 mg, by mouth
- 24 hours to 48 hours after taking mifepristone: misoprostol, 800 μg, buccally
- 7 days to 14 days after taking mifepristone: follow-up to verify that expulsion has been completed

Expected side effects include heavier bleeding than regular menses and passing clots within a few hours after administration of misoprostol. Cramping and pain also are expected before and at time of expulsion. Misoprostol also causes prostaglandin effects, such as nausea, vomiting, diarrhea, dizziness, headache, fevers, and chills.[25] Complications are described later.

Pain management

In most instances, pain from medication abortion can be managed with oral nonsteroidal anti-inflammatory drugs (NSAIDs). If a patient cannot tolerate NSAIDs, acetaminophen is an option, although it has been shown less effective than NSAIDs.[59] Mild opioid analgesics can be helpful for significant cramping or severe pain.

Follow-up after medication abortion

Follow-up 7 days to 14 days after mifepristone can be done by clinical examination, ultrasound, or serum human chorionic gonadotropin (hCG) measurement.

Methods of Abortion: Uterine Aspiration Abortion

Uterine aspiration involves evacuation of the contents of the uterus through a cannula, with manual vacuum aspiration using a hand-held, hand-activated, plastic 60-mL aspirator, or with electric vacuum aspiration.[40] The appropriate-sized cannula is usually chosen based on the GA. **Fig. 1** demonstrates a procedural tray set-up for a uterine aspiration procedure. **Fig. 2** reviews steps for uterine aspiration abortion.

Pain management

Supportive verbal communication and techniques, such as guided imagery, can help in reducing anxiety and pain.[60] A heating pad during or after the procedure is also helpful. Pharmacologic methods can include local anesthetic in a paracervical block, NSAIDs, narcotics, and anxiolytics.[39,61] Paracervical block using lidocaine is effective and recommended to decrease pain with cervical dilation and uterine aspiration.[39,62] Premedication with NSAIDs has been shown to decrease pain during and after the procedure.[39,63] Premedication with narcotic analgesics provide pain relief but may be less effective than NSAIDs.[61] Anxiolytics may decrease anxiety related to the procedure and may cause amnesia for some women but do not affect pain.[61,64]

MANAGEMENT OF MEDICATION AND UTERINE ASPIRATION ABORTION COMPLICATIONS

First-trimester abortion is an exceedingly safe procedure. Abortion has a major complication rate of less than 0.5%.[15] Complications related to medication abortion in the office setting are low. Medication abortions provided within family medicine clinics suggest success rates of approximately 96%.[12,65] A recent systematic review that evaluated complications among 16 office-based studies conducted in the United

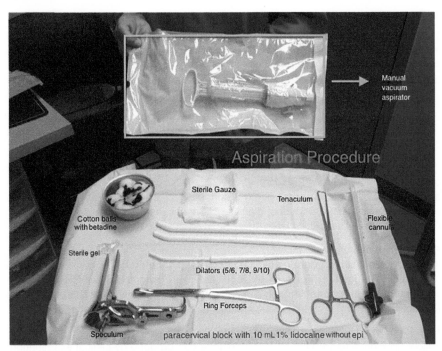

Fig. 1. Typical tray set up for uterine aspiration.

States and Canada found a very low complication rate related to first-trimester uterine aspiration.[66] Similarly, evidence from several family medicine clinics demonstrated that 96.2% of uterine aspiration procedures were successfully completed without complications.[65] Among family medicine residents performing first-trimester aspiration procedures, the complication rate was 1.0%.[31] Although abortion remains safer than full-term delivery throughout the first and second trimesters, the rate of complications increases with increasing GA, by approximately 38% by each additional week after 8 weeks.[40]

Medication Abortion Complications

A majority of problems encountered for medication abortion include incomplete abortion, continuing pregnancy, bleeding, and, rarely, infection.[12,65]

Incomplete Abortion

Incomplete abortion can be managed with a repeat dose of misoprostol. The dosage and dosing intervals for misoprostol for incomplete medication abortion have not been well established. A comprehensive review of first-trimester spontaneous abortion recommends a single dose of 600 μg oral or 400 μg sublingual misoprostol for incomplete abortion.[67] Repeat misoprostol may not be feasible when bleeding is heavy. Heavy bleeding often requires a uterine aspiration procedure or management in the hospital setting.

Continuing pregnancy

Two studies reporting on medication abortion in family medicine settings suggest continuing pregnancy ranges from 1.5% to 1.7%, although overall continuing

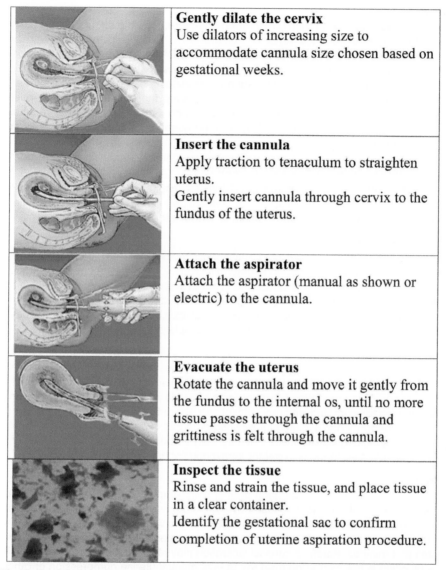

	Gently dilate the cervix Use dilators of increasing size to accommodate cannula size chosen based on gestational weeks.
	Insert the cannula Apply traction to tenaculum to straighten uterus. Gently insert cannula through cervix to the fundus of the uterus.
	Attach the aspirator Attach the aspirator (manual as shown or electric) to the cannula.
	Evacuate the uterus Rotate the cannula and move it gently from the fundus to the internal os, until no more tissue passes through the cannula and grittiness is felt through the cannula.
	Inspect the tissue Rinse and strain the tissue, and place tissue in a clear container. Identify the gestational sac to confirm completion of uterine aspiration procedure.

Fig. 2. Steps for aspiration abortion. (*Adapted from* TEACH Training. Using MVA and EVA equipment. In: Early abortion training workbook, chapter 5: uterine aspiration procedure. Available at: https://www.teachtraining.org/training-tools/early-abortion-training-workbook/. Accessed March 15, 2017; with permission.)

pregnancy in national clinical trials were lower, at approximately 0.7%.[12,25,65] Ongoing pregnancy requires repeat medication or an aspiration procedure.

Bleeding

Uterine bleeding is expected among all women undergoing a medication abortion. Heavy bleeding, soaking through 2 maxipads per hour for more than 2 hours in a row, may be a sign of incomplete abortion (discussed previously).

Infection

Infection associated with medication abortion is rare. Patients should contact their provider if they experience fever of 100.4°F or higher. Clinicians must also be aware of a rare infection that can occur more than 24 hours after taking misoprostol, caused by *Clostridium sordellii*. In these cases, patients often complain of abdominal pain or general malaise, such as weakness, nausea, vomiting, or diarrhea, and infrequently present with fever.[68] Rarely these infections have been associated with death. Suspicion of infection with *Clostridium sordellii* requires prompt medical attention and admission to the hospital for intravenous antibiotics and monitoring.

First-Trimester Aspiration Abortion Complications

A majority of problems encountered in first-trimester aspiration abortions within the office setting include retained products of conception, uterine infection, and bleeding related to cervical laceration, perforation, or uterine atony.

Retained products of conception

When the aspirated tissue does not appear consistent with GA, an ultrasound, if available in clinic, should be performed to determine if there is a persistent gestational sac, which requires reaspiration. If ultrasound is not available, the provider may decide to follow serum quantitative β-hCG gonadotropin levels, drawn the day of the procedure and repeated 48 hours to 72 hours later. A fall of at least 50% from the serum hCG day-of-procedure level indicates the procedure is complete.[69]

Uterine infection

Endometritis after surgical abortion is reduced with the routine use of prophylactic antibiotics, such as doxycycline, and the use of sterile instruments.[39,61,70] If patients are properly counseled regarding the symptoms of pelvic infection, they usually present early enough to be treated with oral antibiotics in the outpatient setting. An ultrasound should be performed to evaluate for retained products of conception, and, if present, aspiration should be performed. Patients with evidence of systemic involvement should be admitted to the hospital for intravenous antibiotics and monitoring.

Bleeding

Excessive bleeding occurring during or after a first-trimester office uterine aspiration procedure is most commonly caused by uterine atony or cervical tears.[40] Source of bleeding should be ascertained via inspection of the vagina and cervix. Hemostasis of the cervix can usually be achieved with compression with a ring forceps for 2 minutes to 3 minutes. Rarely, a cervical laceration may require placement of sutures. If the bleeding is believed to be from the uterus, manual uterine compression or other uterotonic administration, such as methergine or misoprostol, may be necessary. Perforation is an uncommon complication of first-trimester aspiration abortion. It is often asymptomatic and self-healing, occurring in the midline or fundal location. Perforations can be managed with observation and close-follow-up.[70]

ABORTION AFTERCARE

Once completion of the abortion is confirmed, no further follow-up is necessary. Patients should be advised about expected symptoms as well as about symptoms that could indicate a complication.[39,70] Although a range of emotions after an abortion is common, a majority of patients report feeling relief, and many studies have disproved the myth that abortion leads to negative mental health consequences.[71–73]

Postabortion Contraception

All patients should receive postabortion contraceptive information and provision before leaving the primary care clinic.[39] Fertility returns quickly after an abortion, in as few as 8 days after medical abortion and 10 days after uterine aspiration.[74–76] Ideally patients should start contraception within 7 days after a medication abortion or uterine aspiration abortion if they desire preventing a subsequent pregnancy.[77] All contraceptive methods are safe to use after uncomplicated abortion. An IUD or implant may be placed immediately after a first-trimester uterine aspiration procedure or at the time that a medication abortion is confirmed complete.[74,78] Providing methods at the time of abortion, rather than requiring follow-up, increases contraceptive uptake and reduces the risk for unintended pregnancy.[78]

SUMMARY

Unintended pregnancy is commonly encountered in the primary care setting. Approximately half of patients choose to terminate their pregnancies. Primary care providers need to know how to counsel, assess, and provide care to patients seeking abortion. Health care providers should familiarize themselves with the specific regulations related to abortion in their state. First-trimester abortion care, provided either with medication or a uterine aspiration, is exceedingly safe and is feasibly offered in the outpatient clinical setting. Complications, although rare, should be managed appropriately. All patients seeking abortion should receive contraceptive counseling and initiate a postprocedure contraceptive plan at time of the procedure or the follow-up visit.

REFERENCES

1. CDC. National Ambulatory Medical Care Survey: 2013 State and National Summary Tables. Available at: https://www.cdc.gov/nchs/data/ahcd/namcs_summary/2013_namcs_web_tables.pdf. 2016. Accessed March 13, 2017.
2. American College of Obstetricians and Gynecologists. ACOG Committee Opinion number 313, September 2005. The importance of preconception care in the continuum of women's health care. Obstet Gynecol 2005;106(3):665–6.
3. Farahi N, Zolotor A. Recommendations for preconception counseling and care. Am Fam Physician 2013;88(8):499–506.
4. Johnson K, Posner SF, Biermann J, et al. Recommendations to improve preconception health and health care–United States. A report of the CDC/ATSDR Preconception Care Work Group and the Select Panel on Preconception Care. MMWR Recomm Rep 2006;55(RR-6):1–23.
5. Gavin L, Moskosky S, Carter M, et al. Providing quality family planning services: recommendations of CDC and the U.S. Office of Population Affairs. MMWR Recomm Rep 2014;63(RR-04):1–54.
6. Finer LB, Zolna MR. Declines in unintended pregnancy in the United States, 2008-2011. N Engl J Med 2016;374(9):843–52.
7. Jones RK, Jerman J. Abortion incidence and service availability in the United States, 2014. Perspect Sex Reprod Health 2017;49(1):17–27.
8. Raymond EG, Grossman D, Weaver MA, et al. Mortality of induced abortion, other outpatient surgical procedures and common activities in the United States. Contraception 2014;90(5):476–9.
9. Jones RK, Jerman J. Population group abortion rates and lifetime incidence of abortion: United States, 2008-2014. Am J Public Health 2017;107(12):1904–9.

10. Jerman J, Jones R, Onda T. Characteristics of U.S. abortion patients in 2014 and changes since 2008. New York: Guttmacher Institute; 2016.

11. Jatlaoui TC, Ewing A, Mandel MG, et al. Abortion surveillance - United States, 2013. MMWR Surveill Summ 2016;65(12):1–44.

12. Prine L, Shannon C, Gillespie G, et al. Medical abortion: outcomes in a family medicine setting. J Am Board Fam Med 2010;23(4):509–13.

13. Prine LW, Lesnewski R. Medication abortion and family physicians' scope of practice. J Am Board Fam Pract 2005;18(4):304–6.

14. Westfall JM, Sophocles A, Burggraf H, et al. Manual vacuum aspiration for first-trimester abortion. Arch Fam Med 1998;7(6):559–62.

15. Upadhyay UD, Desai S, Zlidar V, et al. Incidence of emergency department visits and complications after abortion. Obstet Gynecol 2015;125(1):175–83.

16. Zane S, Creanga AA, Berg CJ, et al. Abortion-related mortality in the United States: 1998-2010. Obstet Gynecol 2015;126(2):258–65.

17. Roe v. Wade, 410 U.S. 113 (1973).

18. The Departments of Labor and Health, Education, and Welfare Appropriation Act of 1977, Pub L No. 94-439, 94th Congress (1976). Available at: http://uscode.house.gov/statutes/pl/94/439.pdf. Accessed March 26, 2017.

19. Planned Parenthood v. Casey, 505 U.S. 833 (1992).

20. Nash E, Gold RB, Ansari-Thomas Z, et al. Policy trends in the states: 2016. New York: Guttmacher Institute; 2017.

21. Sedgh G, Bearak J, Singh S, et al. Abortion incidence between 1990 and 2014: global, regional, and subregional levels and trends. Lancet 2016;388(10041):258–67.

22. WHO. Unsafe Abortion: Global and regional estimates of the incidence of unsafe abortion and associated mortality in 2008. 6th edition. Geneva (Switzerland): World Health Organization; 2011.

23. Weitz TA, Taylor D, Desai S, et al. Safety of aspiration abortion performed by nurse practitioners, certified nurse midwives, and physician assistants under a California legal waiver. Am J Public Health 2013;103(3):454–61.

24. Barnard S, Kim C, Park MH, et al. Doctors or mid-level providers for abortion. Cochrane Database Syst Rev 2015;(7):CD011242.

25. Mifeprex [package insert]. New York: Danco Laboratories; 2016.

26. American College of Obstetricians and Gynecologists. Practice bulletin no. 143: medical management of first-trimester abortion. Obstet Gynecol 2014;123(3):676–92.

27. Summit AK, Casey LM, Bennett AH, et al. "I don't want to go anywhere else": patient experiences of abortion in family medicine. Fam Med 2016;48(1):30–4.

28. Wu JP, Godfrey EM, Prine L, et al. Women's satisfaction with abortion care in academic family medicine centers. Fam Med 2015;47(2):98–106.

29. Nothnagle M, Sicilia JM, Forman S, et al. Required procedural training in family medicine residency: a consensus statement. Fam Med 2008;40(4):248–52.

30. Kelly BF, Sicilia JM, Forman S, et al. Advanced procedural training in family medicine: a group consensus statement. Fam Med 2009;41(6):398–404.

31. Paul M, Nobel K, Goodman S, et al. Abortion training in three family medicine programs: resident and patient outcomes. Fam Med 2007;39(3):184–9.

32. Summit AK, Gold M. The effects of abortion training on family medicine residents' clinical experience. Fam Med 2017;49(1):22–7.

33. Brahmi D, Dehlendorf C, Engel D, et al. A descriptive analysis of abortion training in family medicine residency programs. Fam Med 2007;39(6):399–403.

34. Singer J. Options counseling: techniques for caring for women with unintended pregnancies. J Midwifery Womens Health 2004;49(3):235–42.

35. Joffe C. The politicization of abortion and the evolution of abortion counseling. Am J Public Health 2013;103(1):57–65.
36. Cockrill K, Upadhyay UD, Turan J, et al. The stigma of having an abortion: development of a scale and characteristics of women experiencing abortion stigma. Perspect Sex Reprod Health 2013;45(2):79–88.
37. Hanschmidt F, Linde K, Hilbert A, et al. Abortion stigma: a systematic review. Perspect Sex Reprod Health 2016;48(4):169–77.
38. ACGME. ACGME program requirements for graduate medical education in family medicine. 2007. Available at: http://www.acgme.org/acWebsite/downloads/RRC_progReq/120pr07012007.pdf Accessed September 2, 2013.
39. WHO. Safe abortion: technical and policy guidance for health systems. 2nd edition. Geneva (Switzerland): World Health Organization; 2012.
40. Paul M, Lichtenberg ES, Borgatta L, et al. Management of unintended and abnormal pregnancy. Comprehensive abortion care. Oxford, England: Wiley-Blackwell; 2009.
41. Henshaw RC, Naji SA, Russell IT, et al. Comparison of medical abortion with surgical vacuum aspiration: women's preferences and acceptability of treatment. BMJ 1993;307(6906):714–7.
42. Perrucci AC. Decision assessment and counseling and abortion care. 1st edition. Boulder (CO): Rowman & Littlefield Publishers; 2012.
43. Gould H, Foster DG, Perrucci AC, et al. Predictors of abortion counseling receipt and helpfulness in the United States. Womens Health Issues 2013;23(4):e249–55.
44. Richardson C. Misinformed consent: the medical accuracy of state-developed abortion counseling materials. Guttmacher Policy Review 2006;9(4):6–11. Available at: https://www.guttmacher.org/gpr/2006/10/misinformed-consent-medical-accuracy-state-developed-abortion-counseling-materials.
45. Gold RN E. State abortion counseling policies and the fundamental principles of informed consent. Guttmacher Policy Rev 2007;10(4):6–13.
46. Daniels CR, Ferguson J, Howard G, et al. Informed or misinformed consent? Abortion policy in the United States. J Health Polit Policy Law 2016;41(2):181–209.
47. AAP. American Academy of Pediatrics Committee on Adolescence: the adolescent's right to confidential care when considering abortion. Pediatrics 2017;139(2). e20163861, 1-11.
48. AAP. Counseling the adolescent about pregnancy options. American Academy of Pediatrics. Committee on Adolescence. Pediatrics 1998;101(5):938–40.
49. Butler A, Bailey D. The maturity and competence of girls obtaining abortions: are parental involvement laws needed? J Policy Pract 2008;7:58–80.
50. Adler NE, Ozer EJ, Tschann J. Abortion among adolescents. Am Psychol 2003; 58(3):211–7.
51. Guttmacher. State policies in brief: An overview of abortion laws. 2017. Available at: http://www.guttmacher.org/statecenter/spibs/spib_OAL.pdf. Accessed March 13, 2017.
52. Kulier R, Kapp N. Comprehensive analysis of the use of pre-procedure ultrasound for first- and second-trimester abortion. Contraception 2011;83(1):30–3.
53. Raymond EG, Bracken H. Early medical abortion without prior ultrasound. Contraception 2015;92(3):212–4.
54. Guiahi M, Davis A, Society of Family P. First-trimester abortion in women with medical conditions: release date October 2012 SFP guideline #20122. Contraception 2012;86(6):622–30.

55. Benson LS, Micks EA, Ingalls C, et al. Safety of outpatient surgical abortion for obese patients in the first and second trimesters. Obstet Gynecol 2016;128(5): 1065–70.

56. Chen MJ, Creinin MD. Mifepristone with buccal misoprostol for medical abortion: a systematic review. Obstet Gynecol 2015;126(1):12–21.

57. Raymond EG, Shannon C, Weaver MA, et al. First-trimester medical abortion with mifepristone 200 mg and misoprostol: a systematic review. Contraception 2013; 87(1):26–37.

58. Winikoff B, Dzuba IG, Chong E, et al. Extending outpatient medical abortion services through 70 days of gestational age. Obstet Gynecol 2012;120(5):1070–6.

59. Raymond EG, Weaver MA, Louie KS, et al. Prophylactic compared with therapeutic ibuprofen analgesia in first-trimester medical abortion: a randomized controlled trial. Obstet Gynecol 2013;122(3):558–64.

60. Gonzales EA, Ledesma RJ, McAllister DJ, et al. Effects of guided imagery on postoperative outcomes in patients undergoing same-day surgical procedures: a randomized, single-blind study. AANA J 2010;78(3):181–8.

61. Renner RM, Jensen JT, Nichols MD, et al. Pain control in first-trimester surgical abortion: a systematic review of randomized controlled trials. Contraception 2010;81(5):372–88.

62. Tangsiriwatthana T, Sangkomkamhang US, Lumbiganon P, et al. Paracervical local anaesthesia for cervical dilatation and uterine intervention. Cochrane Database Syst Rev 2013;(9):CD005056.

63. Wiebe ER, Rawling M. Pain control in abortion. Int J Gynaecol Obstet 1995;50(1): 41–6.

64. Bayer LL, Edelman AB, Fu R, et al. An evaluation of oral midazolam for anxiety and pain in first-trimester surgical abortion: a randomized controlled trial. Obstet Gynecol 2015;126(1):37–46.

65. Bennett IM, Baylson M, Kalkstein K, et al. Early abortion in family medicine: clinical outcomes. Ann Fam Med 2009;7(6):527–33.

66. White K, Carroll E, Grossman D. Complications from first-trimester aspiration abortion: a systematic review of the literature. Contraception 2015;92(5):422–38.

67. Blum J, Winikoff B, Gemzell-Danielsson K, et al. Treatment of incomplete abortion and miscarriage with misoprostol. Int J Gynaecol Obstet 2007;99(Suppl 2): S186–9.

68. Aldape MJ, Bryant AE, Stevens DL. Clostridium sordellii infection: epidemiology, clinical findings, and current perspectives on diagnosis and treatment. Clin Infect Dis 2006;43(11):1436–46.

69. van der Lugt B, Drogendijk AC. The disappearance of human chorionic gonadotropin from plasma and urine following induced abortion. Disappearance of HCG after induced abortion. Acta Obstet Gynecol Scand 1985;64(7):547–52.

70. National Abortion Federation. Clinical Policy Guidelines. Washington, DC 2016. Available at: https://prochoice.org/wp-content/uploads/2016-CPGs-web.pdf. Accessed March 27, 2017.

71. Biggs MA, Rowland B, McCulloch CE, et al. Does abortion increase women's risk for post-traumatic stress? Findings from a prospective longitudinal cohort study. BMJ Open 2016;6(2):e009698.

72. Rocca CH, Kimport K, Gould H, et al. Women's emotions one week after receiving or being denied an abortion in the United States. Perspect Sex Reprod Health 2013;45(3):122–31.

73. Munk-Olsen T, Laursen TM, Pedersen CB, et al. Induced first-trimester abortion and risk of mental disorder. N Engl J Med 2011;364(4):332–9.

74. Benson J, Andersen K, Brahmi D, et al. What contraception do women use after abortion? An analysis of 319,385 cases from eight countries. Glob Public Health 2018;13(1):35–50.
75. Boyd EF Jr, Holmstrom EG. Ovulation following therapeutic abortion. Am J Obstet Gynecol 1972;113(4):469–73.
76. Schreiber CA, Sober S, Ratcliffe S, et al. Ovulation resumption after medical abortion with mifepristone and misoprostol. Contraception 2011;84(3):230–3.
77. Curtis KM, Jatlaoui TC, Tepper NK, et al. U.S. selected practice recommendations for contraceptive use, 2016. MMWR Recomm Rep 2016;65(4):1–66.
78. Bednarek PH, Creinin MD, Reeves MF, et al. Immediate versus delayed IUD insertion after uterine aspiration. N Engl J Med 2011;364(23):2208–17.

Female Athlete Triad

Jennifer P. Daily, MD[a,b,*], Jessica R. Stumbo, MD[a,b]

KEYWORDS

- Female • Female athlete • Amenorrhea • Menstrual dysfunction • Bone health
- Stress fractures • Disordered eating • Low energy availability

KEY POINTS

- The female athlete triad is a metabolic injury. It includes an imbalance between input and output, which can be intentional or inadvertent.
- The goal is to restore the balance between energy intake and energy expenditure by increasing energy in and/or decreasing exercise energy expenditure.
- Prevention and early recognition of the triad are key.

INTRODUCTION

The female athlete triad (triad) is an intertwined relationship between energy availability (EA), bone health, and menstrual dysfunction that can be observed in physically active girls and women. The American College of Sports Medicine (ACSM) initially defined the triad in 1992, and in 1997 the first position statement was published by the ACSM.[1] In 2007, an updated position statement was released, and in 2014, the Female Athlete Triad Coalition released a consensus statement on treatment and return to play.[2–4] The triad is a severe injury that has both short-term and long-term impacts on individual health. Prevention and early recognition should be the cornerstones of management.

DEFINITION

The definition of the triad has evolved over time. The classic terminology included disordered eating, amenorrhea, and osteoporosis. It is now described as a metabolic injury that can be observed in physically active girls and women. The most recent definition contains the following parameters[2–4]:

- Low EA with or without disordered eating
- Menstrual dysfunction
- Low bone mineral density (BMD)

Disclosure: The authors have nothing to disclose.
[a] KentuckyOne Health, University of Louisville, Louisville, KY, USA; [b] Department of Family and Geriatric Medicine, Centers for Primary Care, University of Louisville, 215 Central Avenue, Suite 205, Louisville, KY 40208, USA
* Corresponding author. Department of Family and Geriatric Medicine, Centers for Primary Care, 215 Central Avenue, Suite 205, Louisville, KY 40208.
E-mail address: jennifer.daily@louisville.edu

Prim Care Clin Office Pract 45 (2018) 615–624
https://doi.org/10.1016/j.pop.2018.07.004
0095-4543/18/© 2018 Elsevier Inc. All rights reserved.

The components of the triad exist on a continuum. It is not uncommon for an individual to initially only have 1 or 2 of the components, at which time she may be referred to as having pretriad, and it is critical to intervene to prevent progression.

In 2014, the International Olympic Committee introduced a new phrase to describe the concept of energy imbalance, which is called relative energy deficiency of sports, which refers to a syndrome of impaired physiologic function instead of a triad. The relative energy deficiency results in impaired functions within the realms of metabolic rate, menstrual function, bone health, immunity, protein synthesis, and cardiovascular health. It broadens the definition to include both boys and women and girls and women.[5]

Low Energy Availability

EA is a balance between the energy put in the body (ie, nutrition) and the energy the body expends (physical activity and natural metabolic processes). Low EA refers to a negative balance between energy intake and energy output. Some athletes decrease EA by restricting intake whereas others expend more energy. This imbalance is not always intentional. Athletes progressing to a higher level of demand can inadvertently get into a negative energy balance due to increased energy expenditure without realizing the need for additional intake.[2–4]

Low EA is obvious when there is a body mass index (BMI) less than 17.5 kg/m^2 or less than 85% of expected body weight in adolescents. When overt signs of low EA are absent, determining the EA is more complex but can be calculated as energy intake (kcal) minus exercise energy expenditure (kcal) divided by fat-free mass (kg). Estimates of exercise energy expenditure are subject to bias because they are largely a self-reported measure. Recruiting the help of an experienced dietician can be useful in calculating these assessments. Low EA is defined as less than 30 kcal/kg of fat-free mass per day and below this value is where negative implications, such as menstrual dysfunction and bone health issues, begin to arise. Optimal EA is greater than 45 kcal/kg of fat-free mass per day.[2–4,6,7]

Menstrual Dysfunction

Menstrual irregularities exist on a spectrum from eumenorrhea to functional hypothalamic amenorrhea (FHA). Girls and women presenting with amenorrhea, either primary or secondary, warrant investigation for an underlying etiology because FHA is a diagnosis of exclusion.[2–4] When the body is in a negative energy balance, it suppresses reproductive physiology to conserve energy.[3,4] Menstrual irregularities often can be one of the first clues that a female athlete is in an energy crisis. Return of normal menses can take more than 1 year after improvement of the EA.[7]

Low Bone Mineral Density

The ACSM as well as the International Society of Clinical Densitometry (ISCD) have published definitions for low BMD and osteoporosis in children, adolescents (**Box 1**), and premenopausal women (**Box 2**). The z score is used in the interpretation, not the T score that is traditionally used in postmenopausal women. The ACSM defines low BMD as a z score that is less than −1.0 in female athletes in weight-bearing sports instead of less than or equal to −2.0 as defined by the ISCD because they expect bone mass should be higher in these athletes. Therefore, a BMD z score between −1.0 and −2.0 warrants further evaluation and attention.[2,8–11]

> **Box 1**
> **Definition of osteoporosis and low bone mineral density in children and adolescents (ages 5–19)**
>
> Diagnosis of osteoporosis in children and adolescents requires the presence of both a clinically significant fracture history and BMD z score less than or equal to −2.0. The term, osteoporosis, should not be used without a clinically significant fracture history.
>
> - A clinically significant fracture history is 1 or more of the following:
>   ○ Vertebral compression fracture
>   ○ Two of more long bone fractures by the age of 10
>   ○ Three or more long bone fractures at any age up to age 19 years
>
> - The term, osteopenia, should not appear in pediatric DXA reports. In absence of a clinically significant fracture history, low BMD is the preferred term for pediatric DXA reports when the BMD score is less than or equal to −2.0.
>
> - A BMD z score greater than −2.0 does not preclude the possibility of skeletal fragility and increased fracture risk.
>
> [a] ACSM defines low BMD as z score that is less than −1.0 in female athletes in weight-bearing sports.[2]
> *Data from* Gordon CM, Leonard MB, Zemel BS. 2013 Pediatric position development conference: executive summary and reflections. J Clin Densitom 2014;17:219–24.

EPIDEMIOLOGY

Although the triad is typically believed to affect competitive athletes, it can have an impact on athletes at all experience levels, from recreational to the elite. The triad is a spectrum of diseases, therefore making determining exact prevalence difficult.[10–12]

Gibbs and colleagues[11] performed a systemic review of 65 studies in exercising women to identify prevalence estimates of the triad. There is a paucity of literature regarding all 3 of the components of the triad and, in this systemic review, only 9 studies reported the prevalence of all 3 components, with a range of 0% to 15.9%. The majority of the existing research looks at each individual component of the triad (menstrual dysfunction, disordered eating, and low BMD). The study found the prevalence of any 1 component of the triad 16% to 60% and any 2 components 2.7% to 27%.[12]

Gibbs and colleagues[11] also examined the prevalence of all 3 triad components in lean sport versus nonlean sport athletes. As expected, the prevalence of all 3 components as well as each individual component was higher in lean sport athletes compared with nonlean sport athletes.

> **Box 2**
> **Definition of low bone mineral density and osteoporosis in premenopausal women**
>
> - A BMD z score of less than or equal to −2.0[a] is defined as below the expected for age.
>
> - A BMD z score greater than −2.0 is within the expected range for age.
>
> - Osteoporosis is diagnosed if there is a BMD z score of less than or equal to −2.0 plus secondary causes of osteoporosis.
>
> [a] ACSM defines low BMD as z score that is less than −1.0 in female athletes in weight-bearing sports.[2]
> *Data from* Lewiecki EM, Gordon CM, Baim S, et al. International Society for Clinical Denistometry 2007 adult and pediatric office positions. Bone 2008;43:1115–21; and Gordon CM, Leonard MB, Zemel BS. 2013 Pediatric position development conference: executive summary and reflections. J Clin Densitom 2014;17:219–24.

More studies using consistent definitions of each component of the triad are needed to more accurately determine the prevalence.

RISK FACTORS

Any girl or woman involved in exercise, organized or not, is at increased risk for the triad. Sports and activities that emphasize leanness, aesthetics, and/or endurance place girls and women at greatest increased risk.[2,11] Commonly implicated activities include swimming, diving, running, dancing, gymnastics, cheerleading, rowing, and wrestling.

Risk factors for low EA include restriction of dietary energy intake, prolonged periods of exercise, vegetarians, and those who limit the types of food they consume. Risk factors for stress fractures include low BMD, menstrual dysfunction, dietary deficiencies, training errors, biomechanical abnormalities, and genetic predisposition.[2,13]

SCREENING

Few data exist regarding the effectiveness of screening; however, early detection of athletes at risk for the triad is critical.[14] It is currently recommended to screen female athletes during the preparticipation or annual health examination. Furthermore, when girls and women present for evaluation of related issues, such as fatigue, declining performance, recurrent injury, or illnesses, triad components should be inquired about. Screening can be done with a triad-specific questionnaire, such as the Triad Consensus Panel Screening Questionnaire, published in *British Journal of Sports Medicine* and *Current Sports Medicine Report* in 2014, as follwos[2–4,15]:

- Have you ever had a menstrual period?
- How old were you when you had your first period?
- When was your most recent menstrual period?
- How many periods have you had in the past 12 months?
- Are you presently taking any female hormones (estrogen, progesterone, or birth control pills)?
- Do you worry about your weight?
- Are you trying to or has anyone recommended that you gain or lose weight?
- Are you on a special diet or do you avoid certain types of foods or food groups?
- Have you ever had an eating disorder (ED)?
- Have you ever had a stress fracture?
- Have you ever been told you have low bone density (osteopenia or osteoporosis)?

Screening should occur at both the high school and collegiate levels. Identification of any 1 of the components of the triad should prompt further investigation for the other components.[2–4,15]

PHYSICAL EXAMINATION

Physical examination of many athletes with the triad are often normal or may only demonstrate low BMI or bradycardia. Relying on the vital signs of an athlete as a means of risk stratification can be difficult because many athletes have a lower resting heart rate and bradycardia is common. In extreme cases, however, the examination may demonstrate abnormalities, as seen in **Box 3**.[16]

> **Box 3**
> **Physical examination findings, often associated with more severe cases**
>
> - Lanugo
> - Hair loss
> - Dry skin
> - Brittle hair and nails
> - Callus or abrasion on back of hand (from induced vomiting)
> - Bradycardia
> - Swollen parotid glands
>
> *Adapted from* Sundgot-Borgen J. Disordered eating. In: Ireland ML, Nattiv A, editors. The female athlete. Philadelphia: Saunders; 2002. p. 242–3; with permission.

EVALUATION

The work-up and evaluation of an athlete who has signs and symptoms of the triad include laboratory testing, cardiac work-up, and imaging.

Laboratory Tests

Female athletes presenting with menstrual dysfunction, disordered eating, EDs, or other risk factors for the triad should undergo laboratory testing to evaluate for an underlying etiology, such as thyroid disease, or complications, such as electrolyte disturbances. A more extensive laboratory evaluation may be indicated depending on the clinical features of each case (**Box 4**).

Not all studies have recommended testing leptin in the initial evaluation; however, it is suggested by several centers that treat athletes with severe EDs, including the (McCallum Place, St. Louis, MO, USA). Leptin is an adipocyte-secreted hormone that plays a key part in energy homoeostasis. Advances in leptin physiology have established that the key role of this hormone is to signal EA in energy-deficient states. Studies in animals and humans have shown that low concentrations of leptin are partly if not fully responsible for starvation-induced changes in neuroendocrine axes, including low reproductive, thyroid, and insulinlike growth factor (IGF) hormones. Disease states, such as exercise-induced hypothalamic amenorrhea and anorexia nervosa, are also associated with low concentrations of leptin and a similar spectrum of neuroendocrine abnormalities.[17] Having a baseline level of leptin at the initiation of treatment can be helpful to determine the extent of malnutrition. Following this level longitudinally can be useful for the athlete as well as the care team to demonstrate overall improvement and response to treatment.

Cardiac Work-Up

An electrocardiogram is recommended in athletes with suspected triad because metabolic dysregulation can increase an athlete's risk for cardiac arrhythmias.

Imaging

Dual-energy x-ray absorptiometry (DXA) is the gold standard to measure BMD. The 2014 Female Athlete Triad Coalition consensus statement divides those that should get DXA scans into 3 categories, namely, those considered at high risk, those considered at moderate risk, and those with a history of previous fracture.[3] See **Box 5** for details.

Box 4
Laboratory testing

- Basic laboratory tests
  - Pregnancy test
  - Complete blood cell count with differential
  - Comprehensive metabolic panel
  - Ferritin
  - Thyroid-stimulating hormone
  - Lipid panel
  - Vitamin D
  - Leptin
- Other possible laboratory tests
  - T3 and T4
  - Iron, total iron-binding capacity
  - Erythrocyte sedimentation rate
  - Vitamin B_{12} and folic acid
  - Magnesium
  - Phosphorous
  - Albumin
  - Total protein
  - Urinalysis
  - Luteinizing hormone/follicle-stimulating hormone
  - Estradiol
  - Testosterone
  - Prolactin
  - Bone turnover markers
    - Alkaline phosphatase
    - Osteocalcin
    - Procollagen type I carboxyl terminal propeptide
    - Procollagen type I nitrogen terminal propeptide
    - Hydoxyproline
    - Deoxypyridinoline
    - Pyridinoline
    - N-telopeptide
    - C-telopeptide

Data from Refs.[2,7,15]

Although DXA, a 2-D assessment of a 3-D structure, is the gold standard for evaluation of BMD, newer technology that provides a 3-D evaluation is available, however not as readily accessible. Axial quantitative CT and peripheral quantitative CT can measure bone geometry, bone mass, and volumetric BMD specific to trabecular and cortical bone. Early studies are promising that this imaging provides a more accurate reflection of the bone health in triad and pretriad individuals.[7,10,12]

CLINICAL MANAGEMENT

Treatment of the triad requires a multidisciplinary approach. **Box 6** lists potential team members useful in the management of the triad. Key components of treatment include modification of diet as well as exercise behaviors to increase EA and restore a positive energy balance.[12]

Nonpharmacologic

Restoring energy balance is critical and can be done by increasing intake or decreasing output. Translating that into clinical practice can be challenging.

Box 5
Who should get dual-energy x-ray absorptiometry scans for bone mineral density testing?

- High-risk athletes are those who have greater than or equal to 1 of the following risk factors:
  - History of *Diagnostic and Statistical Manual of Mental Disorders* (Fifth Edition) diagnosis of ED
  - BMI less than or equal to 17.5 kg/m^2, less than 85% estimated weight, or recent weight loss of greater than or equal to 10% in 1 month
  - Menarche greater than or equal to 16 years of age
  - Current or history of fewer than 6 menses over the past 12 months
  - Two prior stress fractures, 1 high-risk stress fracture, or a low-energy nontraumatic fracture
  - Prior z score of less than −2.0 (after at least 1 year from baseline DXA)

- Moderate-risk athletes are those with greater than or equal to 2 of the following risk factors:
  - Current or history of disordered eating for 6 months or greater
  - BMI between 17.5 and 18.5, less than 90% estimated weight, or recent weight loss of 5% to 10% in 1 months' time
  - Menarche between 15 and 16 years of age
  - Current or history of 6 to 8 menses over the past 12 months
  - One prior stress reaction/fracture
  - Prior z score between −1.0 and −2.0 (after at least 1-year interval from baseline DXA)

- Athletes with the following:
  - History of greater than or equal to 1 nonperipheral or greater than or equal to 2 peripheral long bone traumatic fractures (nonstress), with associated 1 or more moderate-risk or high-risk factors
    - Depends on the age at which the fracture occurred and the magnitude of the trauma that caused the fracture (ie, low impact vs high impact).
  - Athletes on medications for 6 months or greater that may have an impact on bone health, including oral contraceptives, intramuscular contraceptives, and oral prednisone, also should be considered for DXA testing.

Data from De Souza MJ, Nattiv A, Joy E, et al. 2014 Female Athlete Triad coalition consensus statement on treatment and return to play of the female athlete triad: 1st International Conference held in San Francisco, California, May 2012 and 2nd International Conference held in Indianapolis, Indiana, May 2013. Br J Sports Med 2014;48:289–309.

Nutrition

A dietician with training and interest in sports nutrition is crucial to helping the female athlete overcome the negative energy balance. Nutritional education, counseling, and monitoring are sometimes all that is required to reverse the energy deficiency, especially when the energy imbalance was inadvertent.[6] A study published in the *Clinical Journal of Sports Medicine* in 2014 found that dancers with disordered eating displayed lower levels of nutritional knowledge, and this was believed to have an impact on BMI.[18] This finding emphasized the necessity of educating athletes on the importance of adequate nutrition.

Mental health

Cases of disordered eating or EDs require professional mental health evaluation and management by health care providers with an expertise in EDs. These providers need to have an appreciation for the mental as well as physical demands of an individual's sport.[6] Athletes suffering from acute anorexia nervosa often have associated depression, rigidity, weight phobia, and a preoccupation with thoughts related to food and eating.[19] These associated thoughts make treatment difficult, and placing the athlete on a written contract is often necessary to ensure that they follow the treatment guidelines determined by the care team. The written contract provides accountability for the athlete to attend therapy sessions, office visits, and weigh-ins. The contract is often

---

Box 6
Multidisciplinary team

- Health care provider
  - Team physician
  - Primary care provider
  - Endocrinologist
- Psychiatrist
- Psychologist
- Sports dietician
- Athletic trainer
- Parents
- Coaches
- Athlete

---

specific to the particular athlete and can vary based on the severity of the case. Cognitive behavioral therapy is also an effective psychotherapy for EDs.

Weight and resistive training

Replacing cardiovascular training with weight and resistive training is recommended by the American Physical Therapy Association to reduce energy expenditure and increase BMD. Introducing a new form of exercise results in skeletal adaptations due to new loading patterns that ultimately are beneficial for bone strength.[7] Plyometrics also can be beneficial, however should be avoided when recovering from a stress fracture.[7]

Pharmacologic

No medication (or pharmacologic therapy) has been shown consistently effective in treatment of the triad. Additional research is needed to provide evidence-based pharmacologic treatment recommendations.[12] The Triad Consensus Panel recommends pharmacologic options be considered if there is lack of response to nonpharmacologic treatments for at least 1 year or if new fractures develop during nonpharmacologic management.[3]

Oral contraceptive pills

In the past, oral contraceptive pills (OCPs) were frequently prescribed to restore normal menses. Research regarding OCPs has had contradictory outcomes, with some studies showing a benefit to bone health, others showing a decrease in BMD, and some no change.[7,12] This approach also does not address the multitude of other hormonal factors that likely contribute to the underlying physiologic dysregulation/disturbance.[12] Initiating OCPs also results in the loss of the natural marker for when a girl or woman regains optimal energy balance.

Bisphosphonates

Bisphosphonates are commonly used in postmenopausal women for the treatment of osteoporosis because they reduce bone turnover. Limited evidence regarding use of bisphosphonates in premenopausal women exists and the studies that have been done are conflicting. Another barrier to use of bisphosphonates in this age group is that long-term effects of bisphosphonates are unknown and, due to their long half-life, they have potential teratogenic effects on a developing fetus.[7] Bisphosphonate therapy in young women with the triad should be executed only by or in consultation with a board-certified endocrinologist or specialist in metabolic bone diseases, and this is done on a case-by-case basis if all nonpharmacologic treatments have failed. It must be emphasized that the aforementioned pharmacologic therapies are not currently approved by the Food and Drug Administration for increasing BMD or for fracture reduction in young or adult athletes.[3]

Vitamins and minerals

Calcium-rich foods and vitamin D intake should be encouraged and optimized. There is no consensus as to the optimal calcium dosage; however, the ACSM recommends between 1000 mg/d and 1300 mg/d and of vitamin D recommends at least 600 IU/d.[3,7,20]

Future treatment options

Recombinant leptin as well as IGF-I are potential treatments for individuals with amenorrhea and anorexia nervosa as well as FHA. A limiting factor in the use of leptin is a potential side effect of weight loss. Ongoing studies are evaluating various dosing regimens to address this unwanted side effect.[7,12]

RETURN TO PLAY

Although awareness of the triad has increased since the first position statement in 1997, no standardized clearance or return to play guidelines exist. The 2014 Triad consensus statement recommends a risk stratification approach that optimizes the athlete's health while minimizing the risk of injury and illness. Furthermore, they developed a risk stratification protocol for care of the triad athlete, including a worksheet to aid physicians and the entire care team in the risk assessment.[3] Once the risk score is calculated, clearance recommendations ranging from full clearance to restriction from all activities can be determined. Athletes in moderate-risk and high-risk categories should be placed under a written contract with goals and parameters that must be met prior to return to activity. Future research is needed to assess the impact of this risk stratification on return to play as well as the athlete's bone health.[3]

PREVENTION

Prevention of the triad is key and this starts with increased awareness. The entire health care team, athletic administrators, coaches, and parents as well as athletes should have education regarding identification of risk factors for the triad as well as the 3 components of the triad. Knowing and understanding the components of the triad are critical to being able to recognize it early as well as implanting measures to prevent its occurrence. When a risk factor and/or component of the triad is identified, providers are obligated to initiate further evaluation to limit progression and future metabolic insult.[2,15,20]

In conclusion, the triad is a complex condition with short-term and long-term consequences that take a team-based approach to effectively manage.

USEFUL RESOURCES

http://www.femaleathletetriad.org—information for athletes, parents, and coaches regarding the triad

www.mccallumplace.com—eating disorder center in St. Louis, St. Louis, MO, USA

REFERENCES

1. Otis C, Drinkwater B, Johnson M, et al. ACSM position stand: the female athlete triad. Med Sci Sports Exerc 1997;29(5). i–ix.
2. Nattiv A, Loucks AB, Manore MM, et al. American college of sports medicine position stand. The female athlete triad. Med Sci Sports Exerc 2007;39:1867–82.
3. De Souza MJ, Nattiv A, Joy E, et al. 2014 Female athlete triad coalition consensus statement on treatment and return to play of the female athlete triad: 1st international conference held in San Francisco, California, May 2012 and 2nd International Conference held in Indianapolis, Indiana, May 2013. Br J Sports Med 2014;48:289–309.
4. Joy E, De Souza MJ, Nattiv A, et al. 2014 Female athlete triad coalition consensus statement on treatment and return to play of the female athlete triad. Curr Sports Med Rep 2014;13(4):219–32.
5. Mountjoy M, Sundgot-Borgen J, Burke L, et al. The IOC consensus statement: beyond the female athlete triad—relative energy deficiency in sport (RED-S). Br J Sports Med 2014;48:491–7.
6. Temme KE, Hock AZ. Recognition and rehabilitation of the female athlete triad/tetrad: a multidisciplinary approach. Curr Sports Med Rep 2013;12(3):190–9.
7. Ducher G, Turner AI, Kukuljan S, et al. Obstacles in the optimization of bone health outcomes in the female athlete triad. Sports Med 2011;41:587–607.
8. Lewiecki EM, Gordon CM, Baim S, et al. International society for clinical denistometry 2007 adult and pediatric office positions. Bone 2008;43:1115–21.
9. Gordon CM, Leonard MB, Zemel BS. 2013 Pediatric Position Development Conference: executive summary and reflections. J Clin Densitom 2014;17:219–24.
10. Goolsby MA, Boniquit N. Bone health in athletes: the role of exercise, nutrition, and hormones. Sports Health 2017;9(2):108–17.
11. Gibbs JC, Williams NI, De Souza MJ. Prevalence of individual and combined components of the female athlete triad. Med Sci Sports Exerc 2013;45(5):985–96.
12. Barrack MT, Ackerman KE, Gibbs JC. Update on the female athlete triad. Curr Rev Musculoskelet Med 2013;6:195–204.
13. Gabel KA. Special nutritional concerns for the female athlete. Curr Sports Med Rep 2006;5:187–91.
14. Mencias T, Noon M, Hoch AZ. Female athlete triad screening in national collegiate athletic association division I Athletes: is the preparticipation evaluation form effective? Clin J Sport Med 2012;2:122–5.
15. Waldrop J. Early identification and interventions for female athlete triad. J Pediatr Health Care 2005;19:213–20.
16. Lebrun C. The female athlete triad: what's a doctor to do? Curr Sports Med Rep 2007;6:397–404.
17. Chan J. Role of leptin in energy-deprivation states: normal human physiology and clinical implications for hypothalamic amenorrhoea and anorexia nervosa. Lancet 2005;366:74–85.
18. Wyon M, Hutchings K, Wells A, et al. Body mass index, nutritional knowledge, and eating behaviors in elite student and professional ballet dancers. Clin J Sport Med 2014;24:390–6.
19. Holtkamp K, Herpertz-Dahlmann B, Mika C, et al. Elevated physical activity and low leptin levels co-occur in patients with anorexia nervosa. J Clin Endocrinol Metab 2003;88(11):5169–74.
20. Carlson JL, Golden NH. The female athlete triad. The Female Patient 2012;37:16–24.

Menopause

Beth Potter, MD*, Sarina Schrager, MD, MS, Jessica Dalby, MD,
Emily Torell, MD, Adrienne Hampton, MD

KEYWORDS

- Menopause • Perimenopause • Vasomotor symptoms
- Hormone replacement therapy (HRT) • Genitourinary symptoms of menopause

KEY POINTS

- For women at high risk for endometrial cancer who have a negative endometrial biopsy via pipelle sampling, consider further evaluation with hysteroscopy and directed biopsy.
- Offer levonorgestrel intrauterine system as a first-line treatment of endometrial hyperplasia without atypia as well as for other causes of abnormal bleeding once malignancy is excluded.
- Genitourinary symptoms of menopause is the new term to describe vaginal atrophy and other genital sequelae of menopause.
- There is strong evidence for the efficacy of gabapentin for reduction menopausal hot flashes.
- Hormone therapy is the most effective treatment available for vasomotor symptoms of menopause.

Menopause is a time of transition that is marked for many women by fluctuating physiologic changes that impact quality of life in the short term with vasomotor symptoms, sleep and mood disturbances as well as long-term changes such as genitourinary symptoms and decreased bone density. Natural menopause is defined as the absence of menses for 12 months without a pathologic cause. The average age of menopause is 51.4 years but can vary based on socioeconomic status and current tobacco use.[1]

The diagnosis of perimenopause and menopause may be made without laboratory testing. Women more than 45 years old who are experiencing vasomotor symptoms with irregular menses are assumed to be in perimenopause, and those who have not had menses for more than 12 months are menopausal. No blood work is needed. For women without a uterus, menopause should be based on symptoms alone.[2] For women less than 45 years old who are experiencing menstrual cycle

Disclosure Statement: The authors have nothing to disclose.
Department of Family Medicine and Community Health, University of Wisconsin School of Medicine and Public Health, 1100 Delaplaine, Madison, WI 53715, USA
* Corresponding author.
E-mail address: Beth.Potter@fammed.wisc.edu

Prim Care Clin Office Pract 45 (2018) 625–641
https://doi.org/10.1016/j.pop.2018.08.001
0095-4543/18/© 2018 Elsevier Inc. All rights reserved.

changes along with menopausal symptoms, a serum follicle-stimulating hormone (FSH) level can help with diagnosis. For women who are on hormone therapy, combined contraception, or progesterone only, FSH may play a role in determining menopausal status.[2]

During the perimenopause and menopause transition, women may experience a variety of changes. During the early perimenopausal transition, many women will experience increasing variability in the length of menstrual cycles. In the late perimenopausal transition, most women will have episodes of amenorrhea for greater than 60 days and often experience vasomotor symptoms during this time. This later transition lasts between 1 and 3 years. During the perimenopausal transition and for up to 2 years after menopause, FSH levels continue to increase, whereas estradiol (E2) is declining. The hormone levels then stabilize.[3]

Woman may experience many physiologic changes during this transition:

- Menstrual cycle irregularity
- Fluctuating fertility
- Vasomotor symptoms
- Sleep disturbance
- Depression and anxiety
- Urogenital symptoms, including vaginal dryness
- Sexual dysfunction

PERIMENOPAUSAL BLEEDING

Changes in menstrual bleeding patterns often signal the start of perimenopause, with typical onset for women in their mid-40s and lasting for several years. Abnormal uterine bleeding (AUB) is a common concern in this age group. Primary care providers can readily respond with initial evaluation and treatment strategies, with referral to gynecology specialists as needed for advanced evaluative procedures and surgical management.

When considering the differential diagnosis for irregular menstrual bleeding, a helpful framework is to divide potential causes into the categories of structural abnormalities and nonstructural causes. The acronym PALM-COEIN is useful to recall the principal causes in each category (**Table 1**).[4]

The principal goal in the evaluation of menstrual irregularities is exclusion of malignancy before offering treatment strategies. Although most patients diagnosed with endometrial cancer are postmenopausal, up to 20% of patients with endometrial

Table 1	
Causes of abnormal uterine bleeding in perimenopause	
Structural Abnormalities (PALM)	**Nonstructural Causes (COEIN)**
Polyp	Coagulopathy (eg, vWB)
Adenomyosis	Ovulatory dysfunction
Leiomyoma	Endometrial
Malignancy and hyperplasia	Iatrogenic (eg, IUD)
	Not yet classified

Abbreviation: vWB, von Willebrand Disease.

Data from Munro MG, Critchley HO, Broder MS, et al, Disorders FWGoM. FIGO classification system (PALM-COEIN) for causes of abnormal uterine bleeding in nongravid women of reproductive age. Int J Gynaecol Obstet 2011;113(1):3–13.

cancer are premenopausal. Appropriate evaluation begins with a speculum examination to exclude other causes of bleeding from the vagina or cervix followed by a bimanual examination to palpate the uterus and adnexa for any masses. Laboratory studies may be low yield, but pregnancy must clearly be excluded at the initial evaluation. The clinician can further consider checking a complete blood count and prothrombin time/partial thromboplastin time in the setting of heavy bleeding history and endocrine evaluation with thyrotropin, prolactin, and serum androgens if suspected by history.

Endometrial biopsy is the first-line test in patients with AUB who are older than 45. Endometrial sampling also should be performed in patients younger than 45 years with a history of unopposed estrogen exposure (patients with obesity or polycystic ovary syndrome), failed medical management, and persistent AUB. Options for endometrial sampling include pipelle (office endometrial biopsy), manual or electric vacuum aspiration, sharp curettage, and hysteroscopy-directed biopsy. Although pipelle is likely the best tolerated method, adequate samples may be difficult to obtain, and there is a risk of missing focal disease. A systematic review of 12 studies, including 1029 women with postmenopausal vaginal bleeding, found sample collection failed in 11% of women and resulted in insufficient sampling in 31%.[5] When adequate samples were achieved, pipelle had a sensitivity of 90% for endometrial cancer and 82% for atypical hyperplasia. This evidence suggests that high-risk women may be further evaluated with hysteroscopy and directed biopsy if their pipelle sampling is negative. Risk factors for endometrial cancer are summarized in **Table 2**.

For women who are less than 45 and low risk for endometrial cancer or for those whom refuse a procedure for initial evaluation, a transvaginal ultrasound can be performed to assess for structural abnormalities and to obtain the endometrial thickness for further risk assessment. Cutoffs for endometrial thickness vary by guideline, with the American College of Obstetricians and Gynecologists (ACOG) recommending that normal in postmenopausal women be considered 4 mm or less, whereas the American College of Radiology suggests 5 mm or less.[6,7] Normal values for endometrial thickness are not well defined for premenopausal women, but general recommendations suggest 16 mm or less as a cutoff.[6] However, if bleeding persists, even in the face of normal transvaginal ultrasonography findings, biopsy is an important next step.

Additional endometrial visualization strategies include saline infusion sonohysterography (SIS) and hysteroscopy. These strategies may be necessary if transvaginal ultrasound is suboptimal or indicative of endometrial lesions that require further investigation. SIS consists of infusion of saline into the endometrial cavity followed by performing ultrasonography, which allows for visualization of endometrial irregularities such as polyps, submucosal fibroids, and focal endometrial hyperplasia. SIS has a sensitivity of 96% to 100% and negative predictive value of 94% to 100% for

Table 2	
Patient risk factors for endometrial cancer	
Estrogen Exposure	**Other**
Unopposed estrogen therapy	Age >50
Tamoxifen	HTN
Early menarche	Diabetes
Late menopause	Thyroid disease
Nulliparity/infertility	Family history
Polycystic ovary syndrome	Lynch syndrome
Obesity	

assessing the uterus and endometrium for pathologic condition.[6] Hysteroscopy uses a flexible scope to look through the cervix into the uterus. Pelvic MRI may be a helpful adjunct when transvaginal ultrasound is not adequate and SIS is not tolerated.

Treatment of AUB depends on the diagnosis. Endometrial biopsy results often guide further treatment. Hyperplasia is a precursor to endometrial cancer, and atypical hyperplasia is associated with the greatest risk of conversion to adenocarcinoma or can actually coexist with adenocarcinoma. Atypical hyperplasia typically requires hysterectomy. However, hyperplasia without atypia may be treated medically. Studies show regression of hyperplasia over 6 months when treated with the levonorgestrel intrauterine system (LNG-IUS) or oral progesterone, 10 mg 10 to 14 days per month. A systematic review from 2015 including 766 patients showed the LNG-IUS to be superior to oral progesterone in achieving a therapeutic response and showed a significantly decreased rate of hysterectomy.[8] For acute cessation of heavy bleeding, medical options include conjugated equine estrogen (IV), combined hormonal contraceptive pills (patches or ring) (CHC), medroxyprogesterone acetate, and tranexamic acid.[9] For chronic management of AUB that is appropriate for medical treatment, options include LNG-IUS, CHC, progestin therapy, tranexamic acid, and nonsteroidal anti-inflammatory drugs. Unopposed estrogen should not be used long term due to the increased risk for endometrial cancer. Surgical options, depending on cause, may include dilation and curettage (D&C), endometrial ablation, uterine artery embolization, and hysterectomy. For structural causes, hysteroscopy with D&C, polypectomy, and myomectomy may be options as well.

CONTRACEPTION

Fertility continues to be a concern until menopause. Although rates of conception decline for women in their 40s, unplanned pregnancy may still occur. Rates of abortion in the United States actually increased for women in their 30s and 40s between 2008 and 2014, whereas rates for abortion in women less than 20 significantly decreased during this time period.[10]

No contraceptive method should be limited by age alone. However, as women age, they may develop medical comorbidities that must be considered when prescribing hormonal contraception. Clinicians should refer to the US Medical Eligibility for Contraceptive Use (USMEC) for the safety profile of contraceptive methods in the setting of medical conditions.[11] However, the USMEC does not account for multiple medical conditions that may increase risk beyond that conferred by any single condition. Thus, for women with multiple comorbidities, clinician judgment must be used to assess the individual woman's underlying risk for cardiovascular disease before prescribing hormonal contraceptive options. Of note, emergency contraception can safely be used in women for whom hormonal contraception is otherwise not advised and should be offered.[12]

When to stop using contraception is a common clinical question. The US Selected Practice Recommendations for Contraceptive Use states, "Contraceptive protection is still needed for women aged greater than 44 years if the woman wants to avoid pregnancy."[12] The North American Menopause Society recommends contraception for 12 months after the final menstrual period.[13] However, for women using hormonal contraception, amenorrhea is not a reliable marker of ovarian failure, and other symptoms of menopause may be masked. For women over the age of 50 using progestin-only contraception, FSH may be used to help diagnose menopause. The UK-based National Institute for Health and Care Excellence guidelines recommend measuring FSH 6 weeks apart, and if the measurements are greater than 30, then contraception may be discontinued after 1 year.[2] FSH is not a reliable marker for women using CHC, even during the placebo interval. The UK Faculty of Sexual and Reproductive Health-care (FSRH) recommends stopping most methods at age 55, except for CHC and depo-medroxyprogesterone (DMPA) injections, which they recommend stopping at age 50. After age 50, the risks for ongoing CHC and DMPA use likely outweigh the benefits, and women should be counseled on alternative methods to avoid the increased risk of cardiovascular disease. FSRH offers additional guidance for extended use of intrauterine devices (IUDs) such that women with a copper IUD placed after age 40 can continue use until menopause, and women with a 52-mg LNG-IUS placed after age 45 can continue use until 55.[14] If the LNG-IUS is being used for endometrial protection as opposed to contraception, it should be replaced every 5 years.

MOOD AND SLEEP ISSUES DURING MENOPAUSE

During the menopausal transition, there is a 2-fold increase in the risk of significant depressive symptoms.[15] There is an association with the variability of hormone levels, not the actual levels, and depression scores. Several risk factors are also associated with depression in this transition, including previous history of depression, lower social economic status, stress, and higher body mass index. The longer the reproductive period from start to finish, the lower the risk of developing depression.[16] The treatment of mood disorders includes selective serotonin reuptake inhibitor (SSRI), cognitive behavioral therapy, and low-dose estrogen therapy if appropriate.[15]

Sleep disturbances are much more common with aging, and the prevalence increases during the menopausal transition. The prevalence of sleep disruption varies between 39% and 47% in perimenopause and 35% and 60% in postmenopause.[17] The studies are contradictory regarding the role of vasomotor symptoms and sleep disturbance. Certain health conditions are associated with sleep disturbance, including obesity, obstructive sleep apnea, and restless leg syndrome. Because sleep disturbance can worsen depression and anxiety, it is important to treat if it is contributing to mood symptoms. Estrogen therapy can improve sleep quality. Also, melatonin along with the melatonergic receptor ramelton has been found to increase sleep time and sleep efficiency.[17]

GENITOURINARY SYMPTOMS OF MENOPAUSE

Vulvovaginal symptoms are very common in menopausal women, affecting up to 45% of women after menopause.[18] In 2014, the International Society for the Study of Women's Sexual Health and the North American Menopause Society adopted a new terminology for genitourinary and sexual symptoms of menopause.[19] Previously called vulvovaginal atrophy or atrophic vaginitis, this condition is now described as genitourinary symptoms of menopause (GSM) due to the effect on not only the vaginal mucosa but also the urethra and sexual functioning. In contrast to vasomotor symptoms, which decrease with time after menopause, GSM usually do not become apparent until at least 2 to 3 years after menopause and then continue to worsen as women get older. Although this condition is common in postmenopausal women, only a minority of women know that their symptoms are related to menopause and therefore do not address the issue with their clinicians.[20] Contributing to this problem is the fact that in population-based surveys only about half of clinicians actually talk to women about GSM symptoms.[20,21]

Estrogen regulates vaginal physiology, and when it is withdrawn, after menopause, physical changes occur. The vaginal mucosa becomes thinner and less elastic with a loss of collagen, elastin, and hyaluronic acid.[22] Vaginal rugae decrease, and the vaginal epithelium becomes thinner and can be friable and easily injured. Atrophic vaginitis is an older term used, but implies inflammation due to irritated vaginal mucosa only. Vaginal blood flow decreases as does lubrication during sexual arousal.

GSM can include vaginal symptoms, sexual symptoms, and urinary symptoms (**Table 3**). GSM can have a profound impact on postmenopausal women's quality of life, affecting intimacy, enjoyment of sexual intercourse, sleep, and relationships.[23,24] Physical examination findings include thin, pale vaginal epithelium, a pH greater than 5 (normal pH is 3.5–4.5), and increased parabasal cells on a maturation index (**Fig. 1**).[18,22] A speculum examination may also demonstrate an atrophic cervix with a stenotic os. Exclusion of secondary causes of symptoms would include a complete history looking at possible vaginal preparations that can cause irritation, urinalysis, a wet preparation, and testing for any other sexually transmitted infections.

Treatment of Genitourinary Symptoms of Menopause

Initial treatment of a woman presenting with symptoms of GSM includes recommendations for vaginal lubricants and vaginal moisturizers. Lubricants are used with intercourse, whereas moisturizers can be used regularly. Moisturizers may increase fluid content in the vaginal epithelium. This effect lasts about 3 days. Women can choose between water and silicone-based moisturizers based on tolerability. Another nonhormonal treatment of GSM is vaginal laser treatment. Intravaginal use of either a CO_2 or YAG laser shows promise in treatment of symptomatic GSM, although long-term outcomes are lacking.[26] Laser therapy may remodel vaginal connective tissue and improve glycogen storage. Prasterone, an intravaginal dehydroepiandrosterone preparation, was approved by the Food and Drug Administration (FDA) in November 2016 and has also demonstrated efficacy in treatment of symptomatic GSM and dyspareunia.[27]

Intravaginal estrogen is the mainstay of treatment for GSM. Local estrogen is minimally absorbed systemically and does not promote endometrial growth, so concomitant progesterone supplementation is not necessary.[18,28] Vaginal estrogen preparations come in creams, pills, and a slow release silicone ring, as noted in **Table 4**. There is no evidence that any one preparation is better than the other.[28] Dosing is flexible because the goal is to relieve symptoms. For the cream and the pill, dosing normally starts with daily application until symptoms improve and then weans down to anywhere between 1 and 3 times a week.[18] Ospemifene, a systemic estrogen reuptake modulator, is FDA approved for the treatment of GSM. Ospemifene is well tolerated and indicated for women who cannot tolerate local estrogen.[29] Although there is no evidence of increased rates of recurrence for women who have had estrogen-positive breast cancer using vaginal estrogen, the ACOG recommends using all other treatment options before offering vaginal estrogen to those women.[30]

Table 3 Presenting symptoms of genitourinary symptoms of menopause		
Vulvo-Vaginal Symptoms	**Sexual Symptoms**	**Urinary Symptoms**
Vaginal dryness	Dyspareunia	Dysuria
Burning	Bleeding with intercourse	Urinary frequency
Vulvar irritation	Decreased lubrication with arousal	Recurrent urinary tract
Vaginal discharge		infections
Introital retraction		
Decreased vaginal elasticity		

Data from Refs.[19,22,25]

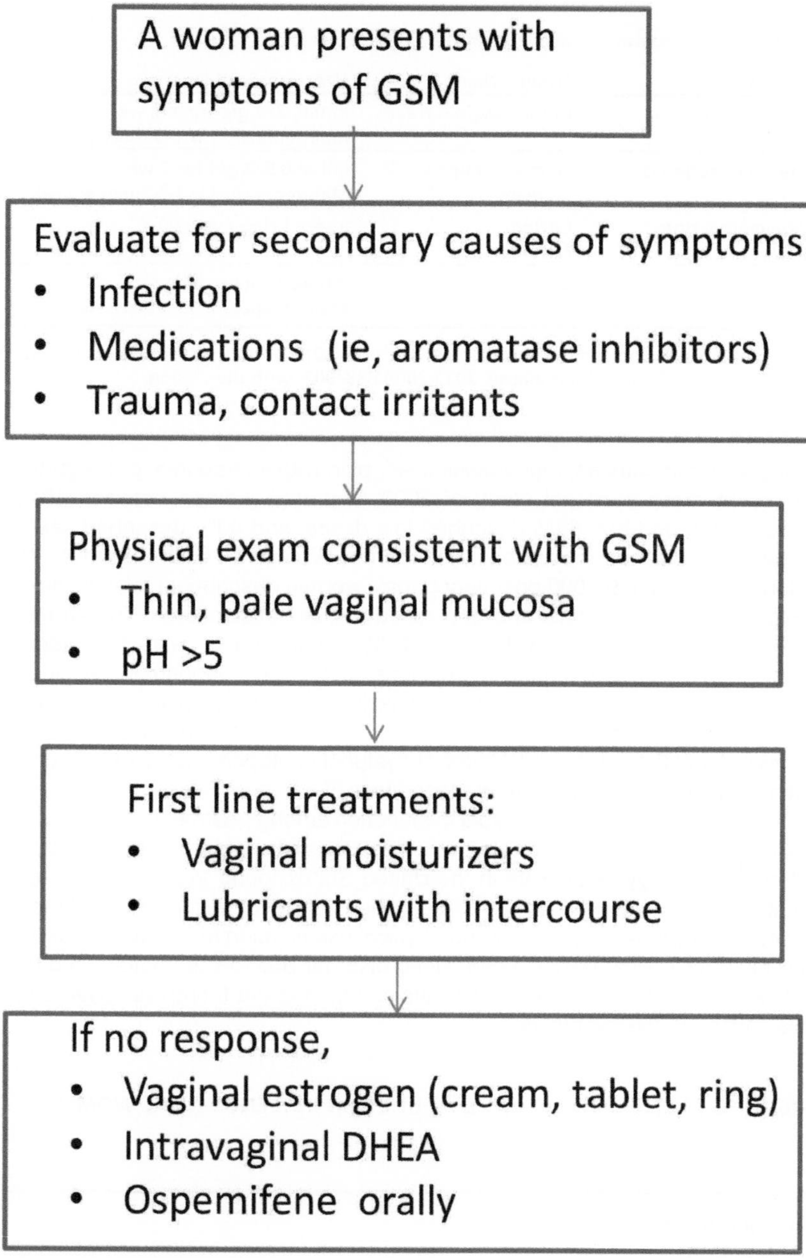

Fig. 1. Management of GSM.

MENOPAUSE AND SEXUAL DYSFUNCTION

Accurate data looking at the prevalence of sexual dysfunction in menopausal women are lacking. Most population-based studies demonstrate high rates of decreasing sexual desire among older women, but it is unclear whether this is due to aging, changing

Table 4
Vaginal estrogen preparations available in the United States

Preparation	Product Name	FDA-Approved Dosing
Estradiol vaginal cream	Estrace vaginal cream	Initial, 2–4 g/d for 1–2 wk Maintenance, 1 g 1–3 times per week
Conjugated estrogen cream	Premarin vaginal cream	Initial 0.5–2 g/d for 3 wk Maintenance, 1 g 1–3 times a week
Estradiol vaginal ring	Estring Femring	Insert 1 ring every 90 d
Estradiol vaginal tablet	Vagifem	Initial, 1 tablet daily for 2 wk Maintenance, 1 tablet twice a week

From Management of symptomatic vulvovaginal atrophy: 2013 position statement of the North American Menopause Society. Menopause. 2013;20(9):888–902; with permission.

psychosocial circumstances, menopause itself, pain with intercourse, or sleep disorders. A recent cross-sectional study of 2000 Australian women between 40 and 65 years of age found that 69% described low desire, and 40% described sexually related personal distress.[31] A subanalysis of the Women's Health Initiative (WHI) that included more than 93,000 postmenopausal women described a relationship between higher rates of insomnia and decreased sexual satisfaction.[32] The Women's Health Across the Nation study followed 1390 women for 5 years to determine when sexual functioning changed in relationship to the menopausal transition.[33] This study demonstrated that women started having decreasing sexual function about 20 months before their final menstrual period. This decrease continued for about a year afterward and then stabilized.[33] Sexual dysfunction appears to be more extreme in women with surgical versus natural menopause.[34]

Despite the high prevalence of sexual dysfunction among postmenopausal women, many clinicians do not ask women about their sexual relationships. One recent survey of 1100 obstetrician-gynecologists in the United States found that only 40% asked women about their sexual problems.[35] The issue is commonly due to a multitude of issues, and a comprehensive history and physical examination may elucidate depression, anxiety, relationship issues, GSM, sleep disorder due to vasomotor symptoms, or female sexual desire disorder.[36] Clinicians can then target therapies based on the probable causes of the dysfunction.

CONTRIBUTING FACTORS TO SEXUAL DYSFUNCTION IN MENOPAUSAL WOMEN

- Dyspareunia due to GSM
- Decreased desire
- Sleep disturbance
- Depression
- Anxiety
- Relationship stresses
- Life changes (ie, children going to college, job changes)

VASOMOTOR SYMPTOMS OF MENOPAUSE

Vasomotor symptoms (ie, hot flashes and night sweats) are common during menopause, affecting between 60% and 80% of women.[37] The cause of vasomotor symptoms is incompletely understood, although E2 and FSH are thought to play an important role because the onset of symptoms coincides with the hormonal changes of the menopausal transition. The mechanism by which FSH and E2 may contribute to vasomotor symptoms is an active area of investigation. There is some evidence that the thermoregulatory zone narrows in symptomatic postmenopausal women and that the administration of E2 can widen this zone.[38,39] In addition, E2 contributes to control of body temperature through peripheral vasodilation leading to greater heat dissipation.[40]

All women experience hormonal changes during the menopausal transition, although not all experience vasomotor symptoms, suggesting there must be other factors involved. Women who are more likely to experience vasomotor symptoms include those who are obese, smokers, African American, have a history of depression/anxiety, or have less than a college education.[37,41] In addition, certain genetic polymorphisms that alter sex steroid hormone activity may predispose some women to vasomotor symptoms.[42,43]

TREATMENT OF VASOMOTOR SYMPTOMS
Hormone Therapy

Systemic estrogen is the most effective therapy for vasomotor symptoms.[13,44,45] In a 2004 Cochrane Review, hormone therapy resulted in a 75% reduction (95% confidence interval [CI], 64.3–82.3) in frequency of hot flashes and a significant reduction in symptom severity (odds ratio, 0.13; 95% CI, 0.07–0.23) compared with placebo.[44] Hormone therapy is available in oral, transdermal, and vaginal preparations. A recent meta-analysis showed that transdermal preparations are the most effective treatment of vasomotor symptoms.[45]

Risks of Hormone Therapy

The risks of hormone therapy differ based on route of administration, dose, duration of use, timing of initiation, and whether progesterone is used.[13]

Contraindications to Hormone Therapy

- Unexplained vaginal bleeding[13]
- Severe active liver disease
- Prior estrogen-sensitive breast or endometrial cancer
- Coronary heart disease
- Stroke or transient ischemic attack
- Untreated hypertension (HTN)
- Dementia
- Active of history of deep vein thrombosis or pulmonary embolism
- Personal history or inherited risk of thromboembolic disease
- Porphyria cutanea tarda
- Hypertriglyceridemia

ENDOMETRIAL HYPERPLASIA

Women with an intact uterus on estrogen therapy should also receive adequate continuous progesterone to prevent endometrial hyperplasia and cancer.[46,47] Micronized progesterone has a more favorable safety profile than synthetic progestin, but its twice daily dosing is a barrier for some women.[48] For women who cannot tolerate the side effects of progesterone (ie, fatigue, dysphoria, and fluid retention), an alternative agent for endometrial protection is the selective estrogen receptor modulator, bazedoxifene.[49,50] The levonorgestrel-releasing intrauterine system has also been used off-label for this purpose and has been shown to be equal or superior to other progesterone formulations in providing endometrial protection.[51,52]

CARDIOVASCULAR AND THROMBOEMBOLIC DISEASE

For women within 10 years of menopause onset or less than 60 years of age without contraindications, the benefits of hormone therapy generally outweigh the risks. A recent Cochrane Review found a lower incidence of coronary heart disease (relative risk [RR] 0.52), reduced all-cause mortality (RR 0.70), and no increased risk of stroke in postmenopausal women on hormone therapy in this age group.[53] Conversely, in women more than 10 years from the onset of menopause or older than 60 years of age, there was an increased risk of stroke (RR 1.21) and no effect on mortality or coronary disease.[53] An increased risk of venous thromboembolism (RR 1.92) and pulmonary embolism (RR 1.81) was found for women of all ages.[53] Cardiovascular risks may be less with transdermal preparations due to avoidance of the first-pass liver effect.[48,54,55] The North American Menopause Society recommends against the use of hormone therapy for women more than 10 years from menopause onset or for women of any age with greater than 10% cardiovascular risk according to the American College of Cardiology/American Heart Association risk calculator.[56]

BREAST CANCER

Postintervention follow-up of the WHI found a significantly increased risk of breast cancer in women taking combined estrogen and progesterone and a nonsignificant reduction in breast cancer risk for those taking estrogen alone.[57] Although the absolute increased risk was small in women taking combined estrogen-progesterone therapy (less than 1 additional case per 1000 person-years of use), these cancers were more likely to be diagnosed at an advanced stage.[57,58] Hormone therapy is contraindicated in women with a history of breast cancer.[13,57]

BILIARY DISEASE

Women taking oral hormone therapy have an approximately 50% increased risk of gallstones and cholecystitis.[57]

MORTALITY

A recent observational follow-up study of the WHI trials found no associated risk of all-cause, cardiovascular, or cancer mortality with hormone therapy during 18 years of follow-up.[59]

DURATION OF HORMONE THERAPY

To minimize the risks of hormone therapy, physicians should prescribe the lowest effective dose for the shortest duration necessary to improve symptoms.[13,60] There is no consensus on the recommended duration of hormone therapy or whether it is best to taper the dose or stop "cold turkey."[13] Approximately half of the women will experience the return of vasomotor symptoms when they stop hormone therapy.[61–63]

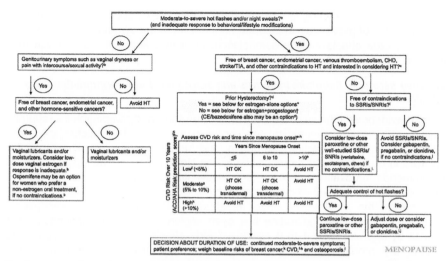

Fig. 2. Approach to pharmacologic treatment of vasomotor symptoms of menopause. CE, conjugated estrogen; CHD, coronary heart disease; CVD, coronary artery disease; HT, hormone therapy. (*From* Manson JE, Ames JM, Shapiro M, et al. Algorithm and mobile app for menopausal symptom management and hormonal/non-hormonal therapy decision making: a clinical decision-support tool from The North American Menopause Society. Menopause 2015;22(3):248; with permission.)

The decision to stop hormone therapy should be individualized based on a patient's symptoms and medical history.[60]

Patient Selection

Fig. 2 outlines an approach to determine if hormone therapy is appropriate for select patients.

Bioidentical Hormones

Bioidentical hormones are structurally identical to those produced by the human body.[64] FDA-approved bioidentical hormones are regulated and monitored for purity and efficacy. These hormones include E2, estrone, and micronized progesterone. In contrast, compounded bioidentical hormones are prepared by a compounding pharmacy that may use multiple hormones that are either untested or unapproved. These preparations are often individualized based on salivary or serum hormone testing and can be administered in nonstandard routes, including subdermal implants, sublingual drops, and troches, raising concerns about consistency in dose and absorption.[65–68] Advocates of compounded hormones claim they are natural, safer, and in some cases more efficacious than conventional therapies, although there is insufficient evidence to support these claims.[48,65–67,69] The American Association of Clinical Endocrinologists, ACOG, and the North American Menopause Society recommend against the use of compounded bioidentical hormones.[13,48,69]

NONHORMONAL THERAPIES
Gabapentin

Several well-designed randomized controlled trials (RCTs) have demonstrated the effectiveness of gabapentin for reduction of hot flash frequency by approximately 2 per day.[70] Doses of 900 mg/d immediate release (divided 3 times a day) and

1800 mg/d of a long-acting formulation have shown the most benefit.[48] The mechanism of action of gabapentin in the treatment of vasomotor symptoms is not well understood. Side effects include somnolence, dizziness, and headache, which may improve after the first few weeks of use.[48]

Selective Serotonin Reuptake Inhibitors and Serotonin-Norepinephrine Reuptake Inhibitors

There is evidence for the efficacy of SSRIs and serotonin and norepinephrine reuptake inhibitor (SNRIs) for menopausal vasomotor symptoms.[71] The mechanism is not clearly understood; however, serotonin and norepinephrine are known to be involved in body temperature regulation.[72] The North American Menopause Society recommends paroxetine, escitalopram, desvenlafaxine, and venlafaxine for the treatment of menopausal vasomotor symptoms.[73] Paroxetine marketed as Brisdelle is currently the only serotonergic agent with FDA approval for menopausal vasomotor symptoms. Paroxetine has been shown to decrease menopausal hot flashes by approximately 1 to 2 per day.[70] Side effects of the serotonergic agents include dry mouth, headache, decreased appetite, nausea, constipation, and insomnia.[70]

Clonidine

Clonidine is a centrally acting alpha-2-adrenergic agonist, which is more effective than placebo at decreasing vasomotor symptoms, although it is less effective than estrogen, SSRI/SNRIs, and gabapentin.[70] A 2006 meta-analysis found an estimated decrease of one hot flash per day with clonidine compared with placebo.[74] The adverse effect profile includes hypotension, headache, nausea, dizziness, sedation, and constipation.[70] With abrupt cessation, rebound HTN can occur.

Table 5
Treatment of vasomotor symptoms

Treatment	Efficacy	Risks/Adverse Events	Notes
Hormone therapy[44,45]	++++	Venous thromboembolism, stroke, cholecystitis, breast cancer, endometrial hyperplasia Dependent on age, dose, route of administration, and duration of use	Transdermal preparations may be more efficacious and carry fewer risks
Gabapentin[78]	+++	Somnolence, dizziness, fatigue	Side effects may abate after a few weeks of use
Paroxetine[70]	++	Dry mouth, headache, decreased appetite, nausea, constipation, and insomnia	Marketed as Brisdelle for menopausal vasomotor symptoms
Venlafaxine[70]	++	Dry mouth, nausea, decreased appetite, constipation, insomnia	
Clonidine[70]	+	Dry mouth, nausea, constipation, insomnia, drowsiness, skin irritation with transdermal form	Sudden cessation can precipitate rebound HTN

+, Up to 24% reduction in symptoms; ++, 25%–49% reduction in symptoms; +++, 50%–74% reduction in symptoms; ++++, 75% or greater reduction in symptoms.

Soy Foods and Supplements

Soy has been found to have weakly estrogenic effects in humans because of the presence of polyphenolic isoflavones, which have estrogen receptor agonist and antagonist activity.[75] A 2016 meta-analysis of 21 RCTs demonstrated a statistically significant improvement in daily hot flashes and vaginal dryness with isoflavone use, from either dietary sources or use of supplements and extracts.[76] Genistein is a particularly promising isoflavone; the authors of a 2013 Cochrane Review note that extracts with high (>30 mg/d) levels of genistein consistently reduced the frequency of hot flashes in 4 RCTs that regrettably could not be pooled for meta-analysis.[77] Research to date has not demonstrated safety concerns related to soy foods, although women are advised to limit whole soy intake to 90 g of soy per day.[75] Synthetic isoflavones have been shown to be associated with increased risk of endometrial hyperplasia (not carcinoma) and subclinical lymphocytopenia.[75]

Table 5 summarizes the pharmacologic treatment options for vasomotor symptoms.

REFERENCES

1. Santoro N, Brockwell S, Johnston J, et al. Helping midlife women predict the onset of the final menses: SWAN, the study of women's health across the nation. Menopause 2007;14(3 Pt 1):415–24.
2. NICE. Menopause: full guideline. United Kingdom: National Institute for Health and Care Excellence (NICE); 2015.
3. Harlow SD, Gass M, Hall JE, et al. Executive summary of the stages of reproductive aging workshop + 10: addressing the unfinished agenda of staging reproductive aging. J Clin Endocrinol Metab 2012;97(4):1159–68.
4. Munro MG, Critchley HO, Broder MS, et al, FIGO Working Group on Menstrual Disorders. FIGO classification system (PALM-COEIN) for causes of abnormal uterine bleeding in nongravid women of reproductive age. Int J Gynaecol Obstet 2011;113(1):3–13.
5. van Hanegem N, Prins MM, Bongers MY, et al. The accuracy of endometrial sampling in women with postmenopausal bleeding: a systematic review and meta-analysis. Eur J Obstet Gynecol Reprod Biol 2016;197:147–55.
6. Bennett GL, Andreotti RF, Lee SI, et al. ACR appropriateness criteria((R)) on abnormal vaginal bleeding. J Am Coll Radiol 2011;8(7):460–8.
7. American College of Obstetricians and Gynecologists. ACOG committee opinion no. 440: the role of transvaginal ultrasonography in the evaluation of postmenopausal bleeding. Obstet Gynecol 2009;114(2 Pt 1):409–11.
8. Abu Hashim H, Ghayaty E, El Rakhawy M. Levonorgestrel-releasing intrauterine system vs oral progestins for non-atypical endometrial hyperplasia: a systematic review and metaanalysis of randomized trials. Am J Obstet Gynecol 2015;213(4):469–78.
9. American College of Obstetricians and Gynecologists. ACOG committee opinion no. 557: management of acute abnormal uterine bleeding in nonpregnant reproductive-aged women. Obstet Gynecol 2013;121(4):891–6.
10. Jerman J, Jones R, Onda T. Characteristics of U.S. Abortion patients in 2014 and changes since 2008. New York: Guttmacher Institute; 2016.
11. Curtis KM, Tepper NK, Jatlaoui TC, et al. U.S. medical eligibility criteria for contraceptive use, 2016. MMWR Recomm Rep 2016;65(3):1–104.
12. Curtis KM, Jatlaoui TC, Tepper NK, et al. U.S. selected practice recommendations for contraceptive use, 2016. MMWR Recomm Rep 2016;65(4):1–66.

13. The NAMS 2017 Hormone Therapy Position Statement Advisory Panel. The 2017 hormone therapy position statement of the North American Menopause Society. Menopause 2017;24(7):728–53.

14. FSRH guideline: contraception for women aged over 40 years (2017). London: Faculty of Sexual & Reproductive Healthcare; 2017. Available at: https://www.fsrh.org/standards-and-guidance/documents/fsrh-guidance-contraception-for-women-aged-over-40-years-2017/.

15. Sassarini DJ. Depression in midlife women. Maturitas 2016;94:149–54.

16. Georgakis MK, Kalogirou EI, Diamantaras AA, et al. Age at menopause and duration of reproductive period in association with dementia and cognitive function: a systematic review and meta-analysis. Psychoneuroendocrinology 2016;73: 224–43.

17. Jehan S, Masters-Isarilov A, Salifu I, et al. Sleep disorders in postmenopausal women. J Sleep Disord Ther 2015;4(5):1–7.

18. Management of symptomatic vulvovaginal atrophy: 2013 position statement of The North American Menopause Society. Menopause 2013;20(9):888–902 [quiz: 903–4].

19. Portman DJ, Gass ML. Genitourinary syndrome of menopause: new terminology for vulvovaginal atrophy from the International Society for the Study of Women's Sexual Health and the North American Menopause Society. Menopause 2014; 21(10):1063–8.

20. Krychman M, Graham S, Bernick B, et al. The women's EMPOWER survey: women's knowledge and awareness of treatment options for vulvar and vaginal atrophy remains inadequate. J Sex Med 2017;14(3):425–33.

21. Simon JA, Kokot-Kierepa M, Goldstein J, et al. Vaginal health in the United States: results from the vaginal health: insights, views & attitudes survey. Menopause 2013;20(10):1043–8.

22. Gandhi J, Chen A, Dagur G, et al. Genitourinary syndrome of menopause: an overview of clinical manifestations, pathophysiology, etiology, evaluation, and management. Am J Obstet Gynecol 2016;215(6):704–11.

23. Kingsberg SA, Wysocki S, Magnus L, et al. Vulvar and vaginal atrophy in postmenopausal women: findings from the REVIVE (REal Women's VIews of Treatment Options for Menopausal Vaginal ChangEs) survey. J Sex Med 2013;10(7): 1790–9.

24. Nappi RE, Kingsberg S, Maamari R, et al. The CLOSER (CLarifying vaginal atrophy's impact on sex and relationships) survey: implications of vaginal discomfort in postmenopausal women and in male partners. J Sex Med 2013;10(9):2232–41.

25. Kim HK, Kang SY, Chung YJ, et al. The recent review of the genitourinary syndrome of menopause. J Menopausal Med 2015;21(2):65–71.

26. Pitsouni E, Grigoriadis T, Falagas ME, et al. Laser therapy for the genitourinary syndrome of menopause. A systematic review and meta-analysis. Maturitas 2017;103:78–88.

27. Labrie F, Archer DF, Koltun W, et al. Efficacy of intravaginal dehydroepiandrosterone (DHEA) on moderate to severe dyspareunia and vaginal dryness, symptoms of vulvovaginal atrophy, and of the genitourinary syndrome of menopause. Menopause 2016;23(3):243–56.

28. Lethaby A, Ayeleke RO, Roberts H. Local oestrogen for vaginal atrophy in postmenopausal women. Cochrane Database Syst Rev 2016;(8):CD001500.

29. McLendon AN, Clinard VB, Woodis CB. Ospemifene for the treatment of vulvovaginal atrophy and dyspareunia in postmenopausal women. Pharmacotherapy 2014;34(10):1050–60.

30. Farrell R. ACOG committee opinion no. 659: the use of vaginal estrogen in women with a history of estrogen-dependent breast cancer. Obstet Gynecol 2016;127(3): e93–6.
31. Worsley R, Bell RJ, Gartoulla P, et al. Prevalence and predictors of low sexual desire, sexually related personal distress, and hypoactive sexual desire dysfunction in a community-based sample of midlife women. J Sex Med 2017;14(5): 675–86.
32. Kling JM, Manson JE, Naughton MJ, et al. Association of sleep disturbance and sexual function in postmenopausal women. Menopause 2017;24(6):604–12.
33. Avis NE, Colvin A, Karlamangla AS, et al. Change in sexual functioning over the menopausal transition: results from the Study of Women's Health Across the Nation. Menopause 2017;24(4):379–90.
34. West SL, D'Aloisio AA, Agans RP, et al. Prevalence of low sexual desire and hypoactive sexual desire disorder in a nationally representative sample of US women. Arch Intern Med 2008;168(13):1441–9.
35. Sobecki JN, Curlin FA, Rasinski KA, et al. What we don't talk about when we don't talk about sex: results of a national survey of U.S. obstetrician/gynecologists. J Sex Med 2012;9(5):1285–94.
36. Iglesia CB. What's new in the world of postmenopausal sex? Curr Opin Obstet Gynecol 2016;28(5):449–54.
37. Gold EB, Colvin A, Avis N, et al. Longitudinal analysis of the association between vasomotor symptoms and race/ethnicity across the menopausal transition: study of women's health across the nation. Am J Public Health 2006;96(7):1226–35.
38. Freedman RR, Krell W. Reduced thermoregulatory null zone in postmenopausal women with hot flashes. Am J Obstet Gynecol 1999;181(1):66–70.
39. Freedman RR, Blacker CM. Estrogen raises the sweating threshold in postmenopausal women with hot flashes. Fertil Steril 2002;77(3):487–90.
40. Charkoudian N, Hart ECJ, Barnes JN, et al. Autonomic control of body temperature and blood pressure: influences of female sex hormones. Clin Auton Res 2017;27(3):149–55.
41. Thurston RC, Joffe H. Vasomotor symptoms and menopause: findings from the Study of Women's Health across the Nation. Obstet Gynecol Clin North Am 2011;38(3):489–501.
42. Rebbeck TR, Su HI, Sammel MD, et al. Effect of hormone metabolism genotypes on steroid hormone levels and menopausal symptoms in a prospective population-based cohort of women experiencing the menopausal transition. Menopause 2010;17(5):1026–34.
43. Schilling C, Gallicchio L, Miller SR, et al. Genetic polymorphisms, hormone levels, and hot flashes in midlife women. Maturitas 2007;57(2):120–31.
44. Maclennan AH, Broadbent JL, Lester S, et al. Oral oestrogen and combined oestrogen/progestogen therapy versus placebo for hot flushes. Cochrane Database Syst Rev 2004;(4):CD002978.
45. Sarri G, Pedder H, Dias S, et al. Vasomotor symptoms resulting from natural menopause: a systematic review and network meta-analysis of treatment effects from the National Institute for Health and Care Excellence guideline on menopause. BJOG 2017;124(10):1514–23.
46. Furness S, Roberts H, Marjoribanks J, et al. Hormone therapy in postmenopausal women and risk of endometrial hyperplasia. Cochrane Database Syst Rev 2012;(8):CD000402.
47. Sjogren LL, Morch LS, Lokkegaard E. Hormone replacement therapy and the risk of endometrial cancer: a systematic review. Maturitas 2016;91:25–35.

48. Cobin RH, Goodman NF. American association of clinical endocrinologists and American college of endocrinology position statement on menopause-2017 update. Endocr Pract 2017;23(7):869–80.

49. Goletiani NV, Keith DR, Gorsky SJ. Progesterone: review of safety for clinical studies. Exp Clin Psychopharmacol 2007;15(5):427–44.

50. Pickar JH, Yeh IT, Bachmann G, et al. Endometrial effects of a tissue selective estrogen complex containing bazedoxifene/conjugated estrogens as a menopausal therapy. Fertil Steril 2009;92(3):1018–24.

51. Somboonporn W, Panna S, Temtanakitpaisan T, et al. Effects of the levonorgestrel-releasing intrauterine system plus estrogen therapy in perimenopausal and postmenopausal women: systematic review and meta-analysis. Menopause 2011;18(10):1060–6.

52. Depypere H, Inki P. The levonorgestrel-releasing intrauterine system for endometrial protection during estrogen replacement therapy: a clinical review. Climacteric 2015;18(4):470–82.

53. Boardman HM, Hartley L, Eisinga A, et al. Hormone therapy for preventing cardiovascular disease in post-menopausal women. Cochrane Database Syst Rev 2015;(3):CD002229.

54. Renoux C, Dell'aniello S, Garbe E, et al. Transdermal and oral hormone replacement therapy and the risk of stroke: a nested case-control study. BMJ 2010;340: c2519.

55. Canonico M, Oger E, Plu-Bureau G, et al. Hormone therapy and venous thromboembolism among postmenopausal women: impact of the route of estrogen administration and progestogens: the ESTHER study. Circulation 2007;115(7): 840–5.

56. Manson JE, Ames JM, Shapiro M, et al. Algorithm and mobile app for menopausal symptom management and hormonal/non-hormonal therapy decision making: a clinical decision-support tool from The North American Menopause Society. Menopause 2015;22(3):247–53.

57. Manson JE, Chlebowski RT, Stefanick ML, et al. Menopausal hormone therapy and health outcomes during the intervention and extended poststopping phases of the Women's Health Initiative randomized trials. JAMA 2013; 310(13):1353–68.

58. Chlebowski RT, Hendrix SL, Langer RD, et al. Influence of estrogen plus progestin on breast cancer and mammography in healthy postmenopausal women: the women's health initiative randomized trial. JAMA 2003;289(24):3243–53.

59. Manson JE, Aragaki AK, Rossouw JE, et al. Menopausal hormone therapy and long-term all-cause and cause-specific mortality: the women's health initiative randomized trials. JAMA 2017;318(10):927–38.

60. ACOG practice bulletin no. 141: management of menopausal symptoms. Obstet Gynecol 2014;123(1):202–16.

61. Ockene JK, Barad DH, Cochrane BB, et al. Symptom experience after discontinuing use of estrogen plus progestin. JAMA 2005;294(2):183–93.

62. Brunner RL, Aragaki A, Barnabei V, et al. Menopausal symptom experience before and after stopping estrogen therapy in the Women's Health Initiative randomized, placebo-controlled trial. Menopause 2010;17(5):946–54.

63. Goff DC Jr, Lloyd-Jones DM, Bennett G, et al. 2013 ACC/AHA guideline on the assessment of cardiovascular risk: a report of the American College of Cardiology/American Heart Association Task Force on practice guidelines. J Am Coll Cardiol 2014;63(25 Pt B):2935–59.

64. Endocrine Society. Bioidentical hormones: position statement. 2006. Available at: https://www.endocrine.org/-/media/endosociety/files/advocacy-and-outreach/position-statements/all/bh_position_statement_final_10_25_06_w_header.pdf?la=en. Accessed October 8, 2017.
65. Sites CK. Bioidentical hormones for menopausal therapy. Womens Health (Lond) 2008;4(2):163–71.
66. Files JA, Ko MG, Pruthi S. Bioidentical hormone therapy. Mayo Clin Proc 2011; 86(7):673–80 [quiz: 680].
67. Cirigliano M. Bioidentical hormone therapy: a review of the evidence. J Womens Health (Larchmt) 2007;16(5):600–31.
68. US Food and Drug Administration. Bio-identicals: sorting myths from facts. 2008. Available at: https://www.fda.gov/forconsumers/consumerupdates/ucm049311.htm. Accessed October 8, 2017.
69. American College of Obstetricians and Gynecologists Committee on Gynecologic Practice, American Society for Reproductive Medicine Practice Committee. Compounded bioidentical menopausal hormone therapy. Fertil Steril 2012;98(2): 308–12.
70. Nelson HD. Menopause. Lancet 2008;371(9614):760–70.
71. Guthrie KA, LaCroix AZ, Ensrud KE, et al. Pooled analysis of six pharmacologic and nonpharmacologic interventions for vasomotor symptoms. Obstet Gynecol 2015;126(2):413–22.
72. Rada G, Capurro D, Pantoja T, et al. Non-hormonal interventions for hot flushes in women with a history of breast cancer. Cochrane Database Syst Rev 2010;(9):CD004923.
73. Nonhormonal management of menopause-associated vasomotor symptoms: 2015 position statement of The North American Menopause Society. Menopause 2015;22(11):1155–72 [quiz: 1173–4].
74. Nelson HD, Vesco KK, Haney E, et al. Nonhormonal therapies for menopausal hot flashes: systematic review and meta-analysis. JAMA 2006;295(17):2057–71.
75. Taylor M. Complementary and alternative approaches to menopause. Endocrinol Metab Clin North Am 2015;44(3):619–48.
76. Franco OH, Chowdhury R, Troup J, et al. Use of plant-based therapies and menopausal symptoms: a systematic review and meta-analysis. JAMA 2016;315(23): 2554–63.
77. Lethaby A, Marjoribanks J, Kronenberg F, et al. Phytoestrogens for menopausal vasomotor symptoms. Cochrane Database Syst Rev 2013;(12):CD001395.
78. Hayes LP, Carroll DG, Kelley KW. Use of gabapentin for the management of natural or surgical menopausal hot flashes. Ann Pharmacother 2011;45(3):388–94.

Bone Health in Women

Jaividhya Dasarathy, MD[a],*, Hallie Labrador, MD, MS[b]

KEYWORDS

- Bone health • Bone mineral density (BMD) • Osteoporosis

KEY POINTS

- Bone health is critically important for overall health of women.
- There are several external factors that are important for bone health that can be modified throughout life.
- Osteoporosis is characterized by decrease in bone mass and increase in fracture risk.

INTRODUCTION

Bone health is critical to the overall health of women. The bony skeleton is an important organ that serves both structural and metabolic functions in addition to being the largest store for calcium and phosphorus in the body.

Healthy bone is strong and adaptable. Bone disease makes bones susceptible to fractures and delays bone healing after injuries. The framework for bone health begins in utero. Bone formation begins before birth and continues to grow and strengthen until approximately age 30. Most bone growth occurs in the first 20 years of life. Loss of bone density begins after the age of 30 and the greatest loss occurs after the age of 50, as women experience menopause (**Fig. 1**).[1]

To play its dual role of support and regulation of calcium and phosphorus metabolism, bone constantly changes. The skeletal system undergoes a process of modeling and remodeling. Specialized cells responsible for breaking down bone (osteoclasts) are coupled with the cells responsible for depositing new bone (osteoblasts).[2] Through the remodeling process, the entire adult skeleton is replaced approximately every 10 years. Imbalances in remodeling can result in both too much bone formation (osteosclerosis) and decreased bone mineral mass (osteoporosis).

Nonmodifiable factors that determine bone health include age, gender, ethnicity, and heredity. There are also several external factors that are important for bone health that can be modified throughout life (**Fig. 2**).

Disclosure: The authors have nothing to disclose.
[a] Department of Family Medicine, Case Western Reserve University, MetroHealth Medical Center, 2500 Metrohealth Drive, Cleveland, OH 44109, USA; [b] Primary Care Sports Medicine Fellowship, North Shore University HealthSystem, University of Chicago Pritzker School of Medicine, 920 North Milwaukee Avenue, Lincolnshire, IL 60069, USA
* Corresponding author.
E-mail addresses: jxd114@case.edu; jdasarathy@metrohealth.org

Prim Care Clin Office Pract 45 (2018) 643–657
https://doi.org/10.1016/j.pop.2018.07.011
0095-4543/18/Published by Elsevier Inc.
primarycare.theclinics.com

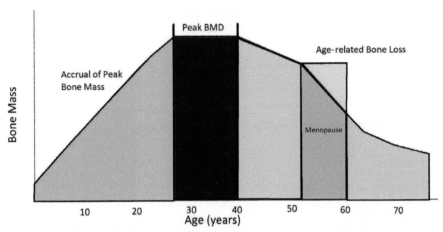

Fig. 1. Bone mass changes through life. (*From* Compston, JE. Review Osteoporosis. Clinical Endocrinology. 1990;33(5):653–82; with permission.)

NUTRITION EFFECTS ON BONE HEALTH

A well-balanced diet promotes bone health. Dietary constituents that play a key role in building and maintaining bone mass include protein, minerals, and vitamins.

Micronutrients

Dietary calcium and vitamin D are critical factors in promoting bone health and preventing bone loss.

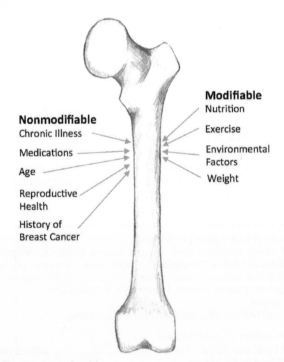

Fig. 2. Factors affecting bone health.

Calcium

Calcium is the single most important nutrient in bone health. Data from the National Health and Nutrition Examination Survey (NHANES)[3] suggest that most Americans older than 3 years do not consume adequate calcium. Current lifestyle and food preferences have resulted in reduced intake of dairy products and other calcium-rich foods. People with lactose intolerance have low bone mass and increased fracture risk.[4] The Institute of Medicine recommends daily adequate intake for calcium, which varies by age and gender[5] (**Table 1**).

Calcium bioavailability is higher with high calcium content foods than calcium supplements. Dairy products are typically the primary dietary sources of calcium. Nondiary sources include Chinese cabbage, kale, turnip, broccoli and other green vegetables, tofu, and calcium-fortified orange juice.[5]

If dietary calcium intake is inadequate, supplements may be necessary. The two main supplemental formulations are calcium carbonate that is absorbed with food and calcium citrate that can be taken with or without food.[6]

Vitamin D

Vitamin D promotes the absorption and utilization of calcium.[7] Dietary sources of vitamin D are limited, with fatty fish the most common source. Vitamin D is produced in the skin when it is exposed to UV light. Many individuals do not get enough vitamin D through sunlight, however, even in sunny climates due to a predominantly indoor life and to sun protection. The Institute of Medicine recommends 600 IU of vitamin D daily for all ages up to 70 and 800 IU after the age of 71.

Vitamin A

Vitamin A plays an important role in bone growth. Excessive vitamin A can, however, trigger an increase in osteoclast activity and may interfere with vitamin D absorption. Excessive vitamin A reduces the overall fracture risk but paradoxically increases the risk of hip fracture.[8]

Other micronutrients, such as phosphorous and magnesium, also contribute to bone strength. Vitamin K is necessary for bone formation and mineralization and vitamin C is required for collagen synthesis. These nutrients are found at sufficient levels in a typical diet and supplements are generally not needed.

Macronutrients

Protein

Optimal protein intake is necessary for developing and maintaining bone mass throughout life. Dietary protein affects bone mass because it is a major component of the structural bone matrix, regulating insulin-like growth factor 1 and affecting

Table 1 Institute of Medicine calcium recommendations for girls and women	
Age (y)	Recommendations (mg/d)
1–3	700
9–18	1300
19–50	1000
>50	1200

From Ross AC, Manson JE, Abrams SA, et al. The 2011 report on dietary reference intakes for calcium and vitamin D from the Institute of Medicine: what clinicians need to know. J Clin Endocrinol Metab 2011;96(1):53–8; with permission.

calcium metabolism. There are conflicting data that high-protein diets may be either detrimental or beneficial to bone health.[9] A recent systematic review showed that high protein intake may have a protective effect on bone mineral density (BMD) in the lumbar spine compared with low intake, but no effect was observed on the hip, femoral neck, or total-body BMD.[9] Despite concerns that the fiber content in plants may limit protein or mineral absorption, there is no measurable difference between plant and animal protein in preventing bone loss.[10]

Dietary fat

Studies show that calcium absorption decreases moderately with increased fat intake. A negative association between saturated fat intake and hip BMD has been reported.[11]

Carbohydrate

High-carbohydrate diets have a detrimental effect on bone health. Diets rich in refined sugars cause increased urinary calcium excretion[12] due to perturbations in renal cell metabolism and insulin signaling. Soft drink or soda consumption may have adverse effects on BMD. Intake of cola, but not other carbonated soft drinks, is associated with lower BMD.[13] Both caffeine and sugar content in the soft drinks have been linked to decreased BMD. Consumption of sports drinks, especially those with a high glucose-to-fructose ratio (eg, Gatorade or Powerade) exert more negative effects on the skeleton than those with a higher fructose-to-glucose ratio (eg, orange juice).[14]

EXERCISE EFFECTS ON BONE
Mechanostat Theory

Bones respond to mechanical forces placed on them and bone strength is correlated to the strain it has to accommodate.[15]

Exercise

Physical activities, especially weight-bearing exercises, increase BMD and reduce fracture risk. The exact age at which women attain peak bone mass is debated; however, most studies indicate that the peak BMD is achieved by early adolescence and young adulthood.[1] Hence, childhood and adolescence are arguably the most important times when interventions affect bone health.

Childhood

Mechanical loading of the bone through exercise is important to achieve a high peak BMD in children. Gains made during childhood can help maintain BMD despite the physiologic bone mineral and strength loss with aging.[16] It is estimated that achieving a 10% higher peak bone mass could delay the development of osteoporosis by approximately 13 years.[17]

Exercise for the osteoporosis prevention should begin in childhood and continue throughout life. The exact amount and type of exercise that is optimal is currently unknown. For bone to adapt to exercise training, however, an overloading force must be applied. Continued adaptation requires progressively increased overload (**Table 2**).[18]

Adulthood

The benefit of exercise for postmenopausal women extends beyond preventing the age-related decline in BMD. Women can increase BMD with high-intensity progressive resistance training regimens, which use exercises that activate muscles against resistance (eg, weightlifting), where the amount of resistance is increased as strength

Table 2	
Exercise principles for osteoporosis prevention	
Exercise Principle	**Examples**
Dynamic exercise	Running, jumping, agility training
Short, intermittent intervals	High-intensity training, drills
Exceed threshold intensity	Sport advancement, increased weights
Variable bone loading	Aerobics, gymnastics, multisport

Data from Kohrt WM, Bloomfield SA, Little KD, et al. American College of Sports Medicine Position Stand: physical activity and bone health. Med Sci Sports Exerc. 2004;36(11):1985–96.

increases. Exercises are performed at a high percentage of maximal amounts of weight that can be lifted.[19] There is also evidence, however, that the response to intense exercise is less robust in postmenopausal than premenopausal women.[20]

Fracture Risk

BMD alone does not determine fracture risk. Low-impact exercise can improve fracture risk without changes in BMD. The Nurses' Health Study found a lower risk of hip fracture in postmenopausal women who reported walking compared with their comparable sedentary peers.[21] This may be due to preservation of fat-free mass or to improved proprioception and balance. Exercise recommendations should be patient-specific and modifications must be made to accommodate for disease states and musculoskeletal limitations of aging.

REPRODUCTIVE EFFECTS ON BONE HEALTH
Menstrual Cycle

Regular menstrual cycles are an important indicator of bone health because they imply normal amounts of estradiol. Estrogen is critically important to bone health. Both women with primary amenorrhea and women with secondary amenorrhea are at risk for decreased BMD and should be evaluated and managed promptly.[22]

In primary ovarian insufficiency, estrogen/progesterone replacement therapy can protect bone strength.

Contraception

Combined estrogen and progestin and progestin-only contraception do not affect bone health.[23] Women using Depo-Provera (DMPA) may lose some bone density transiently but they regain bone density over a short time after stopping DMPA. Although DMPA effect on adolescent bone density loss seems more severe, their loss is reversible with complete recovery within 1 year to 2 years of discontinuation.[24] The Food and Drug Administration added a black box warning on DMPA label cautioning against long-term use (>2 years) in 2004.[25] Several organizations, however, have not incorporated the and Drug Administration warning into their guidelines. DMPA effect on BMD increases the need for counseling and comprehensive education to the patient and importance of shared decision making to decide whether to use it or not and for how long. The effect on BMD and potential fracture risk should not prevent the use of DMPA.[26]

Pregnancy and Lactation

High calcium demand during pregnancy and lactation make women more prone to bone resorption and subsequent osteoporosis. Bone resorption may be reversed after delivery especially if followed by breastfeeding.[27]

Hysterectomy and oophorectomy

Oophorectomy affects calcium metabolism and BMD and increases the risk of fracture in hip and spine and wrist by 54% due to the estrogen and androgen deficiency.[28,29]

MEDICATIONS THAT AFFECT BONE HEALTH

Drug-induced bone loss is a significant health problem, and many physicians are unaware of commonly prescribed medications that cause bone loss and care should be taken when these agents are prescribed (**Table 3**).[30]

BONE HEALTH IN BREAST CANCER SURVIVORS

Breast cancer is common and the mortality for breast cancer has declined in recent years. Breast cancer survivors are at increased risk for future fracture due to several factors:

- Tumor effect on bone
- Breast cancer therapies that affect estrogen metabolism, such as tamoxifen
- Natural menopause
- Glucocorticoids administered with cancer treatments

These risk factors should be taken into consideration when screening and treating breast cancer survivors for osteoporosis.[31]

Table 3
Medication effects on bone health

Medication	Mechanism	Effect/Recommendations
Glucocorticoids	• Stimulates osteoclasts—increased resorption • Induces osteocyte apoptosis • Decreases osteoblast differentiation/function	• Increases fracture risk • 30%–50% of patients receiving glucocorticoids develop fractures • Use bisphosphonates to prevent bone loss
Antiepileptic drugs	• Inactivates vitamin D	• Increases fracture risk • Risk correlated with dosing and duration of treatment • Monitor vitamin D level
Proton pump inhibitors	• Hypochlorhydria decreases calcium absorption • May inhibit osteoclasts—affects bone turnover	• May increase fractures of the hip, wrist, and spine
Aromatase inhibitors	• Lowers estrogen levels—increased bone resorption	• Increased bone loss/fracture risk • Check DXA prior to starting therapy and monitor
Selective seratonin reuptake inhibitors	• Unclear mechanism • Sedation/hypotension may increase falls risk	• Increased fracture risk in hip/nonvertebral sites • Prospective studies needed
Gonadotropin-releasing hormone agonist	• Decreases gonadotropins/estrogen • Induces early menopause	• Increased bone loss • Monitor DXA

Data from Hant FN, Bolster MB. Drugs that may harm bone: mitigating the risk. Cleve Clin J Med 2016;83(4):281–8.

CHRONIC ILLNESS ASSOCIATED WITH BONE HEALTH
Pediatric Chronic Illness

Children with chronic illness such, as celiac disease, type 1 diabetes mellitus (DM), and cystic fibrosis, have impaired bone health. Malabsorption, delayed puberty, hypogonadism, low vitamin D levels, inflammation favoring bone resorption, and glucocorticoid therapy contribute to low BMD. Importantly, fractures can occur even without low mineralization on dual-energy x-ray absorptiometry (DXA) scans.[32]

Optimizing nutrition and vitamin intake, increasing weight-bearing exercise and treating the underlying disease can prevent further bone loss in this group.

Adult Chronic Illness

Diabetes mellitus
Hip fracture risk is increased in both type 1 DM and type 2 DM, whereas BMD is increased in type 2 DM due to hyperinsulinemia and decreased in type 1 DM due to osteoblast inhibition.

Antidiabetic medications can affect bone health and patients preferably should be treated with medications that have positive or neutral effects on bone. Metformin has shown to promote osteogenesis and thiazolidinedione show negative effects on the bone. DDP-4 inhibitors have shown no effects on bone health, and glucagon-like peptide 1 showed mixed results.[33]

Thyroid disorders
Thyroid hormones are necessary for normal skeleton development, and euthyroid status is required for bone accrual and maintenance of adult bone structure and strength. Hyperthyroidism leads to decreased BMD and increased fracture risk. Hypothyroidism, including the subclinical state, can lead to increased fracture risk.[34]

Lupus and rheumatoid arthritis
Patients with lupus are at increased risk of reduced BMD. Vitamin D deficiency, medication use, inhibition of osteoblast formation due to chronic systemic inflammation, and disease severity can contribute to poor bone health. There are no specific guidelines for clinical practice in patients with lupus, but in general guidelines for patients who use chronic glucocorticoids are applied to screen for and treat osteoporosis.[35]

Asthma
A decrease in BMD acquisition in children was associated with high doses of inhaled corticosteroid (ICS) but not low to medium doses of ICSs. In adults, there was a dose-related effect of ICSs on BMD.[36]

Chronic kidney disease
Increasing dietary phosphorus through inorganic phosphate additives in patients with chronic kidney disease has detrimental effects on bone and mineral metabolism.[37]

Chronic liver disease
Osteoporosis and hypovitaminosis are common in patients with chronic liver disease, especially cholestatic diseases like biliary cirrhosis and sclerosing cholangitis.[38]

EFFECTS OF WEIGHT ON BONE HEALTH

Because bone strength is affected by the mechanical load placed on bone,[15] bones that support a heavier load are expected to be stronger. The effect of body mass index on bone health, however, is complicated. There is an increased risk for osteoporosis and fracture in both women who are underweight[39] and who are overweight.[40]

Underweight

Low body weight is a known risk factor for fracture and is incorporated into algorithms that predict fracture risk.[39] Because women with low body mass index often have menstrual abnormalities, it is difficult to determine if risk is related to weight or hormonal effects in premenopausal women.

Overweight/Obesity

Absolute adiposity (subcutaneous adipose tissue) correlated positively and relative adiposity (visceral fat) correlated negatively with bone mass.[41] Bariatric surgeries cause higher BMD deterioration; therefore, more attention is needed to prevent fracture.[42]

ENVIRONMENTAL FACTORS AND BONE HEALTH
Smoking

Tobacco use is inversely related to BMD in women. It has an impact on several factors that contribute to bone health[43]:

- Hormone effects: decreased parathyroid hormone and estrogen, increased cortisol, and adrenal androgens
- Reduced vitamin D levels
- Increased free radicals and oxidative stress
- Reduced blood supply to the bones
- Decreased muscle mass, balance, and neuromuscular performance resulting in increased falls risk
- Tobacco smoke toxicity on bone cells

Active smoking increases the risk of developing osteoporosis and fractures in women, particularly after menopause. Meta-analysis has shown that fracture risk with smoking may be independent from decreases in BMD, indicating a deficit in bone quality.[44]

Data from meta-analyses demonstrate that smokers have double the risk of nonunion after surgical procedures and time to union after fracture compared with nonsmokers.[45]

The relationship between smoking and fracture risk seems to be dose dependent and may be partially reversible with smoking cessation. Meta-analysis shows a significantly increased relative risk of hip fracture in high-dose female smokers (more than 15 cigarettes/d) compared with low-dose smokers and a significant decline in risk in women who had quit for greater than or equal to 10 years.[46]

Lead Exposure

Lead is stored within the bone and prior exposure can cause effects when it gets released into the bloodstream as bone is reabsorbed during menopause. Inhalation of automotive exhaust from leaded gasoline use in early 1970s, drinking water use through lead-soldered plumbing, and handling lead-based paints are the sources of lead exposure. The NHANES III study found a significant inverse association between lead exposure and BMD in white subjects.[47]

Alcohol and Bone Health

Response to alcohol consumption is dose-dependent, with heavy consumption leading to unfavorable outcomes and light consumption providing potential benefits.[48]

BONE HEALTH IN OLDER ADULTS; OSTEOPOROSIS

Osteoporosis is characterized by decrease in bone mass and microarchitectural changes in the bone, which increases fracture risk. Advancing age is the most common risk factor for osteoporosis. In postmenopausal women, osteoporosis is often accelerated due to the loss of the protective effects of estrogen. Osteoporotic fractures are associated with increased risk of disability, nursing home placement, total health care cost, and mortality.[49]

Risk Factors

There are certain modifiable and nonmodifiable risk factors associated with osteoporosis (**Table 4**).

Screening for osteoporosis may help facilitate treatment before fractures occur. Screening techniques use imaging to estimate BMD, which correlates to bone strength. DXA is the validated standard of care technique to measure BMD.[50] Most organizations recommend initiating BMD screening for women at the age of 65 or younger, if they have risk factors. No guidelines have been issued regarding the interval of screening or cessation of screening; however, experts suggest repeating DXA after 2 years of treatment to monitor effects. Because of the limitations of DXA, the World Health Organization Fracture Risk Assessment Tool (FRAX) better predicts fracture risk and is widely used. This application includes an appropriate group of patients for osteoporosis treatment and it calculates a patient's 10-year probability of hip and other major osteoporotic fractures using the individual DXA score as well as clinical risk factors.[51] The FRAX clinical risk factors include age, gender, race, height, weight, prior fragility fracture, and parental history of hip fracture, current smoking, alcohol intake, and long-term use of steroids.

Prevention

Many interventions are used to prevent osteoporosis-related fracture risk. These include vitamin supplements, weight-bearing exercise, tobacco avoidance, moderate alcohol intake, antiresorptive and prodeposition therapy, and avoidance of trip or fall hazards.[52]

Vitamin D and Calcium Supplementation

Supplementation is considered beneficial for fracture prevention. There was recent concern, however, about the efficacy and potential risks of supplementation. The US Preventive Services Task Force recently recommend against the daily supplementation of vitamin D_3 and calcium for the primary prevention of fractures in noninstitutionalized postmenopausal women based on the recent meta-analysis. Some investigators reported increased cardiovascular risk and kidney stones associated with supplementation.[53]

Table 4
Risk factors of osteoporosis

Nonmodifiable	Modifiable
White or Asian race	Sedentary lifestyle
Old age	Smoking
Early menopause	More than 2 drinks/d
Small body frame	Caffeine intake
Family history	Low levels of vitamin D and calcium
History of fracture	Reduced intake of fruits and vegetables

Data from Cosman F, de Beur SJ, LeBoff MS, et al. Clinician's guide to prevention and treatment of osteoporosis. Osteoporos Int 2014;25(10):2359–81.

Pharmacotherapy

Physicians can use osteoporosis risk assessment tools to estimate the absolute fracture risk when considering medications. The FRAX predictions can help guide counseling for patients.[50]

Treatment Guidelines

The National Osteoporosis Foundation recommends initiating pharmacotherapy under the following conditions:

- History of hip or vertebral fractures (regardless of symptoms)
- T-score less than or equal to −2.5 at the femoral neck, total hip, or lumbar spine
- Women greater than age 50 with osteopenia and 10-year hip fracture probability of greater than or equal to 3% or a 10-year major osteoporosis-related fracture of greater than or equal to 20% based on FRAX calculations[43]

Pharmacotherapy Options

There are several pharmacotheapeutic options available for treating osteoporosis and they are effective in reducing the fracture, morbidity and mortality See **Table 5**.

Pharmacotherapy Considerations

Bisphosphonates are first-line antiresorptive medications for osteoporosis. Multiple trials have shown significantly reduced vertebral and nonvertebral fracture risk with these medications within 6 months to 1 year of starting.[54]

Table 5
Pharmacotherapy options for osteoporosis

Medication	Use	Risks
Bisphosphonates	Considered first line	Atypical fractures and bisphosphonate-related osteonecrosis of the jaw—both seen more commonly with >5 y treatment and high doses
Calcitonin	Questionable efficacy Possible pain relief for acute vertebral compression fractures	Possible increased cancer risk
Selective estrogen receptor modulators	Preferred for postmenopausal women with high-risk for breast cancer	Increased thromboembolic events Increased menopausal symptoms
Hormone replacement therapy	Not recommended for osteoporosis but may reduce fracture risk if taken for menopausal symptoms	Increased risk of breast cancer, VTE, and stroke
Human recombinant parathyroid hormone	Anabolic agent can increase BMD	Only approved for 2-y duration Risk of osteosarcoma
RANKL (receptor activator of nuclear factor-κB) ligand inhibitor	Reserved for high-risk women	Hypocalcemia Possible increased infection risk

Data from Cosman F, de Beur SJ, LeBoff MS, et al. Clinician's guide to prevention and treatment of osteoporosis. Osteoporos Int 2014;25(10):2359–81.

- Oral bisphosphonates may be dosed every day, every week, or every month.
- Creatinine clearance less than 30 mL/min is a contraindication to all bisphosphonates.
- Patients with esophageal disorders, history of bariatric surgery, or difficulty remaining upright may benefit from intravenous bisphosphonates.

Although the bisphosphonate-associated risk for osteonecrosis of the jaw is extremely low, it is a primary concern for many patients. Risk of osteonecrosis of the jaw for patients taking osteoporosis doses of bisphosphonate is estimated between 1 in 10,000 and 1 in 100,000 patients per year.[55] Patients should be advised to optimize oral health by completing any necessary oral surgery prior to initiating therapy and maintaining twice-yearly dental cleanings.

Atypical femur fractures are another low but widely feared risk to taking bisphosphonates. Several studies have shown an association between duration of treatment with bisphosphonate and this complication; however, causality has not been shown.[54] Regardless, any complaint of groin and thigh pain in a patient with a history of bisphosphonate exposure should be evaluated to rule out atypical fracture.

Because of concern for these rare adverse events, patients are typically maintained on bisphosphonates for 3 years to 5 years, after which they are stopped. Effects of bisphosphonate on bone can persist even after stopping the medication. Some patients who remain at high risk for fracture may benefit from long-term use[56]:

- Patients with a femoral neck T-score less than −2.5 after 3 year to 5 years of treatment
- Patients with existing vertebral fracture with a somewhat higher T-score
- Patients with a femoral neck T-score greater than −2.0 are unlikely to benefit from continued treatment

Calcitonin was widely used in the past for osteoporosis treatment; however, given newer more effective agents and a potential increased risk of cancer with prolonged treatment, calcitonin is no longer recommended. There may be a role for intranasal calcitonin short term for treatment of pain related to acute vertebral compression fracture.[57]

Selective estrogen receptor modulators may be first-line treatment of women who have contraindications to taking bisphosphonates or women with osteoporosis who also have an increased risk for breast cancer.[58]

- Once-daily dosing
- Efficacy in reducing fractures is less than bisphosphonates
- No known risk to cumulative dosing; however, limited data after 8 years of use
- Not recommended for premenopausal women
- May increase risk of menopausal symptoms and venous thromboembolism, may affect triglycerides in susceptible patients

Hormone replacement therapy does reduce fracture risk by replacing estrogen lost through normal menopause; however, long-term use may cause increased risk for breast cancer, coronary heart disease, venous thromboembolism, and stroke. It is not recommended as first-line osteoporosis treatment.

Human recombinant parathyroid hormone can improve BMD as an anabolic agent; however, cost, administration difficulties, and risks make it a poor choice for first-line therapy.

- Typically used for women who have failed other treatments (eg, recurrent fragility fracture)

- Injected subcutaneously daily
- May be used first line for patients with severe osteoporosis or those who have contraindications to bisphosphonates
- Medication should be discontinued after 2 years.

RANKL ligand inhibitors are not used first line but may be used in patients who are unable to take bisphosphonates.

- Injected subcutaneously every 6 months
- Patients at risk for hypocalcemia should have calcium levels monitored.
- Skin infections may occur and patients should seek treatment of any new skin conditions.

SUMMARY

Strong bones are critical to overall health and quality of life. Although genetic factors play a key role in bone formation, there are several external factors that can be modified to preserve bone health. Diet, exercise, menstrual irregularities, medications, disease states, weight, and environmental factors can all affect fracture risk.

To prevent fractures, patient and physician understanding of bone health needs to improve. This requires a team effort from families, individuals, physicians, the heath care system and community-based organizations, policy makers, and agencies at all levels of government.

REFERENCES

1. Weaver CM, Gordon CM, Janz KF, et al. The National Osteoporosis Foundation's position statement on peak bone mass development and lifestyle factors: a systematic review and implementation recommendations. Osteoporos Int 2016; 27(4):1281–386.
2. Manolagas SC, Parfitt AM. What old means to bone. Trends Endocrinol Metab 2010;21(6):369–74.
3. Bailey RL, Gahche JJ, Lentino CV, et al. Dietary supplement use in the United States, 2003-2006. J Nutr 2011;141(2):261–6.
4. Obermayer-Pietsch BM, Bonelli CM, Walter DE, et al. Genetic predisposition for adult lactose intolerance and relation to diet, bone density, and bone fractures. J Bone Miner Res 2004;19(1):42–7.
5. Ross AC, Manson JE, Abrams SA, et al. The 2011 report on dietary reference intakes for calcium and vitamin D from the Institute of Medicine: what clinicians need to know. J Clin Endocrinol Metab 2011;96(1):53–8.
6. Straub DA. Calcium supplementation in clinical practice: a review of forms, doses, and indications. Nutr Clin Pract 2007;22(3):286–96.
7. Bronner F. Recent developments in intestinal calcium absorption. Nutr Rev 2009; 67(2):109–13.
8. Zhang X, Zhang R, Moore JB, et al. The effect of vitamin A on fracture risk: a meta-analysis of cohort studies. Int J Environ Res Public Health 2017;14(9) [pii: E1043].
9. Shams-White MM, Chung M, Du M, et al. Dietary protein and bone health: a systematic review and meta-analysis from the National Osteoporosis Foundation. Am J Clin Nutr 2017;105(6):1528–43.
10. Wallace TC, Frankenfeld CL. Dietary protein intake above the current RDA and bone health: a systematic review and meta-analysis. J Am Coll Nutr 2017; 36(6):481–96.

11. Corwin RL, Hartman TJ, Maczuga SA, et al. Dietary saturated fat intake is inversely associated with bone density in humans: analysis of NHANES III. J Nutr 2006;136(1):159–65.

12. Lennon EJ, Piering WF. A comparison of the effects of glucose ingestion and NH4Cl acidosis on urinary calcium and magnesium excretion in man. J Clin Invest 1970;49(7):1458–65.

13. Tucker KL, Morita K, Qiao N, et al. Colas, but not other carbonated beverages, are associated with low bone mineral density in older women: the Framingham Osteoporosis Study. Am J Clin Nutr 2006;84(4):936–42.

14. Lorincz C, Manske SL, Zernicke R. Bone health: part 1, nutrition. Sports Health 2009;1(3):253–60.

15. Frost HM. Bone's mechanostat: a 2003 update. Anat Rec A Discov Mol Cell Evol Biol 2003;275(2):1081–101.

16. Johnston CC Jr, Slemenda CW. Peak bone mass, bone loss and risk of fracture. Osteoporos Int 1994;4(Suppl 1):43–5.

17. Hernandez CJ, Beaupre GS, Carter DR. A theoretical analysis of the relative influences of peak BMD, age-related bone loss and menopause on the development of osteoporosis. Osteoporos Int 2003;14(10):843–7.

18. Kohrt WM, Bloomfield SA, Little KD, et al. American College of Sports Medicine Position Stand: physical activity and bone health. Med Sci Sports Exerc 2004; 36(11):1985–96.

19. Xu J, Lombardi G, Jiao W, et al. Effects of exercise on bone status in female subjects, from young girls to postmenopausal women: an overview of systematic reviews and meta-analyses. Sports Med 2016;46(8):1165–82.

20. Bassey EJ, Rothwell MC, Littlewood JJ, et al. Pre- and postmenopausal women have different bone mineral density responses to the same high-impact exercise. J Bone Miner Res 1998;13(12):1805–13.

21. Feskanich D, Willett W, Colditz G. Walking and leisure-time activity and risk of hip fracture in postmenopausal women. JAMA 2002;288(18):2300–6.

22. Rosenfield RL. Clinical review: Adolescent anovulation: maturational mechanisms and implications. J Clin Endocrinol Metab 2013;98(9):3572–83.

23. Lopez LM, Grimes DA, Schulz KF, et al. Steroidal contraceptives: effect on bone fractures in women. Cochrane Database Syst Rev 2014;6:CD006033.

24. Curtis KM, Martins SL. Progestogen-only contraception and bone mineral density: a systematic review. Contraception 2006;73(5):470–87.

25. Administration UFaD. Black box warning added concerning long term use of Depo-Provera Contraceptive Injection. 2004.

26. Committee Opinion No. 602: depot medroxyprogesterone acetate and bone effects. Obstet Gynecol 2014;123(6):1398–402.

27. Karlsson C, Obrant KJ, Karlsson M. Pregnancy and lactation confer reversible bone loss in humans. Osteoporos Int 2001;12(10):828–34.

28. Centers for Disease Control and Prevention. Key Statistics from the National Survey of Family Growth, Atlanta, GA. 2015. Available at: http://www.cdc.gov/nchs/nsfg/key_statistics/h.htm - hysterectomy. Accessed May 28, 2018.

29. Melton LJ 3rd, Khosla S, Malkasian GD, et al. Fracture risk after bilateral oophorectomy in elderly women. J Bone Miner Res 2003;18(5):900–5.

30. Hant FN, Bolster MB. Drugs that may harm bone: mitigating the risk. Cleve Clin J Med 2016;83(4):281–8.

31. Bruyere O, Bergmann P, Cavalier E, et al. Skeletal health in breast cancer survivors. Maturitas 2017;105:78–82.

32. Williams KM. Update on bone health in pediatric chronic disease. Endocrinol Metab Clin North Am 2016;45:433–41.

33. Sundararaghavan V, Mazur MM, Evans B, et al. Diabetes and bone health: latest evidence and clinical implications. Ther Adv Musculoskelet Dis 2017;9(3):67–74.

34. Williams GR, Bassett JHD. Thyroid diseases and bone health. J Endocrinol Invest 2018;41(1):99–109.

35. Ensrud KE, Crandall CJ. Osteoporosis. Ann Intern Med 2017;167(3):ITC17–32.

36. Skoner DP. Inhaled corticosteroids: effects on growth and bone health. Ann Allergy Asthma Immunol 2016;117(6):595–600.

37. Vorland CJ, Stremke ER, Moorthi RN, et al. Effects of excessive dietary phosphorus intake on bone health. Curr Osteoporos Rep 2017;15(5):473–82.

38. Handzlik-Orlik G, Holecki M, Wilczynski K, et al. Osteoporosis in liver disease: pathogenesis and management. Ther Adv Endocrinol Metab 2016;7(3):128–35.

39. De Laet C, Kanis JA, Oden A, et al. Body mass index as a predictor of fracture risk: a meta-analysis. Osteoporos Int 2005;16(11):1330–8.

40. Compston J. Obesity and bone. Curr Osteoporos Rep 2013;11(1):30–5.

41. Dolan E, Swinton PA, Sale C, et al. Influence of adipose tissue mass on bone mass in an overweight or obese population: systematic review and meta-analysis. Nutr Rev 2017;75(10):858–70.

42. Rodriguez-Carmona Y, Lopez-Alavez FJ, Gonzalez-Garay AG, et al. Bone mineral density after bariatric surgery. A systematic review. Int J Surg 2014;12(9):976–82.

43. Cosman F, de Beur SJ, LeBoff MS, et al. Clinician's guide to prevention and treatment of osteoporosis. Osteoporos Int 2014;25(10):2359–81.

44. Bijelic R, Milicevic S, Balaban J. Risk factors for osteoporosis in postmenopausal women. Med Arch 2017;71(1):25–8.

45. Pearson RG, Clement RG, Edwards KL, et al. Do smokers have greater risk of delayed and non-union after fracture, osteotomy and arthrodesis? A systematic review with meta-analysis. BMJ Open 2016;6(11):e010303.

46. Shen GS, Li Y, Zhao G, et al. Cigarette smoking and risk of hip fracture in women: a meta-analysis of prospective cohort studies. Injury 2015;46(7):1333–40.

47. Campbell JR, Auinger P. The association between blood lead levels and osteoporosis among adults–results from the third national health and nutrition examination survey (NHANES III). Environ Health Perspect 2007;115(7):1018–22.

48. Gaddini GW, Turner RT, Grant KA, et al. Alcohol: a simple nutrient with complex actions on bone in the adult skeleton. Alcohol Clin Exp Res 2016;40(4):657–71.

49. In: Bone health and osteoporosis: a report of the surgeon general. Rockville (MD) 2004.

50. World Health Organization. Assessment of Osteoporosis at the Primary Health Care Level scientific group on assessment of Osteoporosis 2004, 2014. Available at: http://www.who.int/chp/topics/Osteoporosis.pdf.

51. Kanis JA, Harvey NC, Johansson H, et al. Overview of fracture prediction tools. J Clin Densitom 2017;20(3):444–50.

52. Cosman F, de Beur SJ, LeBoff MS, et al. Erratum to: Clinician's guide to prevention and treatment of osteoporosis. Osteoporos Int 2015;26(7):2045–7.

53. Lutsey PL, Michos ED. Vitamin D, calcium, and atherosclerotic risk: evidence from serum levels and supplementation studies. Curr Atheroscler Rep 2013; 15(1):293.

54. Andreopoulou P, Bockman RS. Management of postmenopausal osteoporosis. Annu Rev Med 2015;66:329–42.

55. Khan AA, Morrison A, Hanley DA, et al. Diagnosis and management of osteonec-rosis of the jaw: a systematic review and international consensus. J Bone Miner Res 2015;30(1):3–23.
56. Black DM, Bauer DC, Schwartz AV, et al. Continuing bisphosphonate treatment for osteoporosis–for whom and for how long? N Engl J Med 2012;366(22):2051–3.
57. Khosla S, Hofbauer LC. Osteoporosis treatment: recent developments and ongoing challenges. Lancet Diabetes Endocrinol 2017;5(11):898–907.
58. Siris ES, Harris ST, Eastell R, et al. Skeletal effects of raloxifene after 8 years: re-sults from the continuing outcomes relevant to Evista (CORE) study. J Bone Miner Res 2005;20(9):1514–24.

Cancer Survivor Health Needs for Women

Jamal Islam, MD, MS[a],*, George D. Harris, MD, MS[b]

KEYWORDS

• Women • Cancer survivor • Surveillance • Health care needs

KEY POINTS

• The number of women cancer survivors is increasing.
• There is an urgent need for coordinated care by primary care health providers (PCHPs), oncologists, and other specialists.
• PCHPs need to understand the complexity of heath care needs and be familiar with survivorship algorithms.

INTRODUCTION

A cancer survivor is a person with a history of cancer, starting from the time of diagnosis until death, not only those who have completed chemo/radiation therapy and have survived. The number of cancer survivors is increasing due to the increase 5-year survival rate as a result of improvements in early detection and treatment. A cancer survivor's health care needs encompass several domains (medical, psychosocial, informational, and proactive contact)[1] and can be lifelong compared with those for a noncancer patient.

Cancer survivors' health care needs depend on age, type of cancer, stage at detection, and previous treatment—medical (chemotherapies, biologic therapies, or immunotherapies), surgical (curative or palliative procedures), and/or radiation (definitive or palliative) as well as their side effects from treatment and genetic risk factors for recurrence or occurrence of new primary cancers. In addition, clinicians and patients should be aware of the Choosing Wisely campaign and its guidelines to individualize their choices and care.

Cancer survivors require a multidisciplinary team—primary health care providers (PHCPs), surgeons, dietitians, behavioral therapists, psychiatrists, physiotherapists,

Disclosure: The authors have nothing to disclose.
[a] Family Medicine Residency, University of Texas Medical Branch, 302 University Boulevard, Galveston, TX 77550, USA; [b] Department of Family Medicine, WVU Eastern Campus, 2500 Foundation Way, Martinsburg, WV 25401, USA
* Corresponding author.
E-mail address: Jaislam@UTMB.edu

Prim Care Clin Office Pract 45 (2018) 659–676
https://doi.org/10.1016/j.pop.2018.07.005
0095-4543/18/© 2018 Elsevier Inc. All rights reserved.

cardiologists, pulmonologists, nephrologists, and other specialists in addition to oncologists.

PHCPs have a crucial role in the health care team in monitoring cancer recurrence and occurrence, treating side effects of cancer therapies and comorbidities, providing psychosocial interventions, and patient education. PHCPs need to be aware of the complexity of care of cancer survivors and be updated on cancer survivor guidelines.

Cancer survivor health care needs change over the course of a lifetime. Stratifying needs accordingly assists primary care health providers (PCHPs) and other team members in understanding their individual responsibilities. Rodriguez and Zandstra proposed a 3-tier survivor risk stratification in the continuum of cancer survivor care. Tier 1 includes patients with very low risk of complications or relapse: PCHPs can handle most of their health care and psychosocial needs. Tier 2 are those patients with treatment-related complications or with a second malignancy: specialists are required in addition to the PCHP. Tier 3 patients have a high risk of relapse; active indolent or controlled disease; intensive chemotherapy/radiation/Stem Cell Transplant with high risk of sequelae.[2] In this tier, oncologists are actively involved in the care alongside specialists and the PCHP, if needed. Using this proposed framework, each group of clinicians is able to provide continued care for the cancer survivor and decrease the likelihood of losing track of these patients and improve their health care needs.

INCIDENCE, PREVALENCE, AND SURVIVAL RATES

- The number of cancer survivors continues to increase each year due to improved cancer screening, diagnostic measures, and defined treatment regimens.
- By January 1, 2026, it is estimated that the population of cancer survivors will increase to 20.3 million, with approximately 10 million men and 10.3 million women.
- In 2016, in the United States, the 3 most prevalent cancers among female survivors were breast, colorectal, and uterine and the 3 most prevalent cancers among men were prostate, colon and rectum, and melanoma. Approximately 56% of survivors were diagnosed within the past 10 years, with approximately one-half at age 70 years or older.[3]
- According to studies reported in the Choosing Wisely campaign, it is not recommended to screen for breast, colorectal, or prostate cancer in patients who have an estimated life expectancy less than 10 years.[4]

Surveillance after treatment
- On completing active treatment, survivors may not receive the surveillance and monitoring needed or the continued preventive and psychosocial interactions and support required as they age.
- Surveillance falls into 2 main categories—local recurrence and distant recurrence. There is often a lack of clarity about who is responsible for survivorship care delivery. The Institute of Medicine report in 2008 recognized the need of a survivorship care plan for better communication between the oncologist, the patient, and the primary care provider(s) to improve the quality of health care for the cancer survivor.
- The Institute of Medicine noted 4 essential components of survivorship care: (1) prevention of recurrent and new cancers and of other late effects; (2) surveillance for cancer spread, recurrence, and secondary cancers; assessment of medical and psychosocial late effects; (3) intervention for consequences of cancer and its treatment; and (4) coordination between primary and specialty care to meet the health care needs of survivors.[5]

- Even though cancer survivors continue to see an oncology team for follow-up disease surveillance, they also need to be seen by a PCHP for health mainte-nance and management of comorbidities that may or may not be related to cancer diagnosis and treatment.[6]
- Timely and appropriate bidirectional communication between the PCHP and specialists is needed for patient referral for management of comorbidities, symp-toms, and long-term and late effects.[7]
- The PCHP should focus on evidence-based preventive care and the manage-ment of preexisting comorbid conditions; provide an assessment of the patient's overall physical and psychosocial status; make appropriate referrals for psycho-social, rehabilitative, or other specialist care as indicated; and coordinate care, encouraging the inclusion of caregivers, spouses, or partners in patients' survi-vorship care and support.[8]

HISTORY AND PHYSICAL EXAMINATION

- Patients should be educated and counseled about the signs and symptoms of local recurrence.
- Screen cancer survivors for other cancers by adhering to the early detection rec-ommendations from the American Cancer Society.[9]
- Assess survivors for long-term and late effects of their cancer and its treatment at each follow-up visit.[8]

Nonspecific Symptoms

Cancer-related symptoms can occur during treatment or often persist after treat-ment.[10] Cancer-related symptoms associated with both cancer and its treatment are often underdiagnosed and undertreated. The most common symptoms experi-enced by cancer survivors include fatigue, insomnia, neuropathy, and pain.

Fatigue
- The etiology of cancer-related fatigue (CRF) is believed to be related to dysregu-lation in the inflammatory process and in the hypothalamic-pituitary-adrenal func-tion, resulting in a persistent sense of tiredness.
- Assess survivors for fatigue and any causative factors, including anemia, thyroid dysfunction, and cardiac dysfunction, as well as any coexisting symptoms (pain, depression, and insomnia).[10]
- A meta-analysis demonstrated that physical exercise helped reduce CRF; the most effective type or intensity of exercise for the treatment of CRF has not been established.[11]

Insomnia
- Assess for sleep disturbances, snoring, and sleep apnea. If sleep apnea is sus-pected, the patient should be referred to a sleep specialist for a polysomnogram.[8]
- A first-line approach should include nonpharmacologic therapies. Therapies that have demonstrated positive benefit include cognitive behavior therapy and exer-cise, specifically, yoga.[12,13]
- A second-line approach, which can be used in conjunction with cognitive behavior therapy and exercise, is pharmacologic treatments, including hydroxy-zine or melatonin. If further pharmacologic treatment is indicated, however, a short-term benzodiazepine (lorazepam or temazepam) may be helpful for those unable to fall asleep. Longer-acting nonbenzodiazepine hypnotics (zolpidem, za-leplon, and eszopiclone) are helpful for those who experience early morning

awakening. These agents have not demonstrated any short-term or long-term benefits and may cause adverse effects, such as tolerance, withdrawal, sedation, cognitive impairment, light-headedness, and somnolence. As the severity of these symptoms increases, the overall quality of life decreases.[10]
- Another second-line choice for sleep is antidepressants (trazodone, doxepin, and amitriptyline) to initiate and maintain sleep. These medications need to be monitored for hypotension, arrhythmias, hyponatremia, hepatotoxicity, and seizures.

Pain
- Pain may be caused by residual tissue damage from the cancer and/or its therapy. The highest prevalence of severe pain occurs during active treatment and with advanced cancer. Chronic pain, however, can also be linked to the aftermath of curative cancer treatment.[14]
- The pain experienced can be somatic, visceral, or neuropathic in origin, with the most common chronic pain syndromes neuropathic in origin due to surgery, radiation therapy, or chemotherapy. Treatment should be tailored using a combination of opioids, analgesics, physical therapy, interventional procedures, psychosocial interventions, and complementary and alternative modalities.[15]
- When chronic pain develops after breast surgery, thoracotomy, limb amputation, and surgical interventions, it may increase the likelihood of depression and insomnia, which has a negative impact on quality of life.[15] Depression and insomnia should be addressed and treated to improve patient quality of life.
- Management of chronic pain must be integrated and balanced, optimizing quality of life while preventing secondary addiction or other complications related to the therapies used.

New physical findings
- Oral infections and candidiasis may occur as a side effect or consequence of cancer treatment. Certain cancer treatments (chemotherapy, targeted cancer drugs, radiotherapy, and high dose of steroids) can temporarily weaken the immune system by diminishing the number of leukocytes and their various immunologic properties. Treatments include systemic fluconazole and/or localized therapy of clotrimazole lozenges (troches).
- Patients with lymphedema should be referred to a rehabilitation specialist for manual lymphatic drainage and compressive bandaging. Lymphedema has adverse cosmetic and psychosocial consequences and can cause pain, musculoskeletal and neurologic dysfunction, infections, and breathing or swallowing difficulties.[8]
- Alterations or loss of taste may require a referral to a registered dietitian for dietary counseling on how to make food more appealing by adding seasonings and expanding dietary options.
- Hearing loss and vertigo require work-up and referral (tympanometry, pure tone testing, speech reception threshold, and word recognition testing as well as distortion product otoacoustic emissions) to an audiologist and/or otolaryngologist for further evaluation.[8] Patients may require tips on reducing noise exposure and/or a hearing aid.[16]

LABORATORY TESTS, IMAGING, AND OTHER STUDIES

- Ordering laboratory tests and special studies depends on patient symptoms and physical signs. Due to the high incidence of hypothyroidism among patients receiving radiation to head and neck area, a thyroid-stimulating hormone (TSH) test should be ordered within 4 weeks after therapy. If TSH indicates hypothyroid state, then replacement therapy is indicated—L-thyroxine is prescribed and TSH level is tested again 6 weeks later and if normal, then tested annually unless symptoms develop beforehand; if still subtherapeutic, then the L-thyroxine dose is increased and the TSH level assessed 6 weeks later.

- Low-dose CT can be ordered for lung cancer screening. Current National Comprehensive Cancer Network guidelines criteria for recommending low-dose CT are individuals ages 55–74 years (1) who have a history of smoking 30-pack-years or more and are current smokers; (2) who have quit smoking within the past 15 years; and (3) who are 50 years or older and have a history of smoking 20-pack-years or more and have an additional risk, such as prior head and neck cancer.[17]

MEDICAL AND PSYCHOSOCIAL CONCERNS

- During their recovery and post-treatment, cancer survivors' main concern is not returning to normal after treatment. They also have difficulties, such as
  1. Depression
  2. Altered body image
  3. Sexuality
  4. Managing comorbid conditions
  5. Barriers to care
- Depression: among cancer survivors, the estimated prevalence rates of anxiety and depression are 17.9% and 11.6%, respectively.[18] Cancer survivors should be screened for distress, depression, and anxiety and followed with appropriate interventions with medications and/or behavioral therapy.
- Altered body image: cancer survivors should be interviewed for body and self-image concerns. Common body image concerns include those associated with urinary or fecal incontinence, ostomy, alopecia, mastectomy, and lumpectomy.
- Sexuality: cancer survivors should be screened for decreased desire and arousal, alternate sensation in orgasm or anorgasmia, intimacy and relationships, and sexual satisfaction.[19] For women, vasomotor symptoms (night sweats, hot flashes, and flushes) and specific genital symptoms (pelvic pain, vaginal dryness, and vaginal stenosis) should be addressed and treated, if appropriate.
- Managing comorbid conditions: cancer survivors are likely to have comorbid conditions that need to be properly managed, decreasing the potential for other complications or to prevent increased mortality from these sources. Therapies instituted to treat diabetes, hypertension, hyperlipidemia, rheumatologic, and collagen vascular diseases need to be monitored for serious and adverse reactions as well as diminished or exaggerated effects from the various agents used for cancer treatment.
- Barriers to care: there are racial and ethnic disparities in health care that prevent some cancer survivors from receiving the highest level of cancer care or appropriate access to care that lead to disproportionate suffering and poor quality care.[20] Other patients lack access to care because of their geographic location and distance to appropriate treatment facilities. The main barrier for cancer survivors in racial/ethnic minority, low socioeconomic status, and uninsured/underinsured groups continues to be the cost of medical treatment.[21]

TREATMENT-RELATED SIDE EFFECTS

Cancer survivors may undergo 1 or more types of cancer treatment: surgery, radiation therapy, and/or systemic therapy involving chemotherapy, hormonal therapy, immune therapy, and targeted therapy.

Surgical Therapy

- Head and neck cancer survivors: may require referral to a rehabilitation specialist for comprehensive neuromusculoskeletal management. Patients suffering from cervical dystonia or neuropathy should be treated with nerve-stabilizing agents, such as pregabalin, gabapentin, and duloxetine, or referred to a specialist for botulinum toxin type A injections, which can help with muscular pain and spasm control.[8] Patients who have head and neck surgery may experience dysphagia, aspiration, and/or esophageal stricture, resulting in postprandial cough, unexplained weight loss, or pneumonia. PCHPs should refer to a speech-language pathologist for an evaluation of swallowing function, dysphagia, and possible aspiration. If a stricture is suspected, gastroenterology referral is warranted.[8]
- Breast cancer survivors: may develop lymphedema. Arm lymphedema occurs in 20% of women who undergo axillary lymph node dissection and in approximately 6% of women who undergo sentinel lymph node biopsy. Breast cancer survivors also may experience numbness, tingling, or tightness in the chest wall, arms, or shoulders after surgery and/or radiation.[22] Women undergoing mastectomy may opt for breast reconstruction with a saline or silicone implant, a tissue flap, or a combination of these approaches. A recent study found that 57% of women with nonmetastatic disease who received mastectomies underwent reconstructive procedures.[23]
- Rectal cancer survivors: may require colostomy (usually temporary) more frequently than for those with colon cancer.
- Uterine cancer survivors: those patients who underwent pelvic surgery (hysterectomy with oophorectomy) may experience hot flashes, night sweats, atrophic vaginitis, and osteoporosis due to female hormone deficiency. Those undergoing pelvic lymphadenectomy or radiation may experience lower extremity lymphedema.

Pharmacologic Therapy

- Chemotherapy-induced peripheral neuropathy (CIPN) is a prominent dose-limiting toxicity that may begin weeks to months after the initiation of treatment. CIPN often presents with a sensory neuropathy, paresthesia, and pain that develop progressively during the course of treatment. After treatment is completed, CIPN symptoms may resolve, reverse partially, or remain unchanged for years.
- Neuropathy is a common side effect of chemotherapy regimens containing oxaliplatin.[24] Oxaliplatin can cause acute sensory neuropathy characterized by cold-induced paresthesia and muscle cramping sensations, which are dose-dependent and dose-limiting and may progress to chronic sensory neuropathy.[25] Symptoms associated with acute and chronic oxaliplatin neurotoxicity can be reduced by adding venlafaxine, 37.5 mg to 225 mg daily. Intravenous calcium and magnesium have been used for the prevention of CIPN with good results. Gabapentin or pregabalin can also be prescribed to treat CIPN.[26]
- Paclitaxel, a chemotherapy drug, has been associated with an acute pain syndrome—paclitaxel acute pain syndrome (P-APS). This pain syndrome is common and seems associated with the development of peripheral neuropathy with sensory neuropathy symptoms more prominent than motor or autonomic neuropathy symptoms. The sensory symptoms (tingling, numbness, burning, and shooting pain) result in a diffuse aching discomfort in the legs, hips, and lower back; they develop within 1 day to 3 days of drug administration and usually resolve within 7 days. P-APS may also include arthralgia or myalgia likely due to neurologic injury. Patients who have higher P-APS scores (>5 of a total score

of 10) after receiving the first dose of paclitaxel are at greater risk of developing more chronic neuropathy.[27]

- Women with breast cancer receiving chemotherapy with taxanes, which block cell growth by stopping mitosis, may experience neuropathy that can persist long after treatment ends. Anthracyclines and human epidermal growth factor receptor 2 (HER2)-targeted drugs can lead to cardiomyopathy and congestive heart failure. Treatment with aromatase inhibitor, a blocker of estrogen production can cause osteoporosis, myalgia and arthralgia. Tamoxifen, a selective estrogen receptor blocker in breast tissue, prescribed to certain breast cancer survivors may increase risk of endometrial and venous thromboembolism. Some of the drugs used in chemotherapy can cause infertility in women as well as men that may be permanent or temporary.[3]
- Survivors with a history of ototoxic drug exposure (eg, cisplatin cumulative dose >100 mg/m^2) are at risk of chronic, potentially progressive sensorineural hearing loss.[28] Head and neck cancer survivors may experience progressive hearing loss even years after the initial treatment with cytotoxic agents and radiation.[29]

Radiation Therapy

- Patients receiving irradiation of the tissues in the head and neck areas should be monitored for developing or worsening of gastroesophageal reflux disease (GERD), which may prevent the healing of irradiated tissues and thereby increase the risk of head and neck cancer recurrence. The recommended treatment regimens for GERD should be followed and, if the symptoms do not resolve, patients should be referred to gastroenterology specialist.[8]
- Hypothyroidism is a frequent sequela of radiation therapy to the head and neck and can occur as early as 4 weeks and as late as 10 years after treatment.[30] Patients should be screened annually with a TSH level.
- Rectal cancer survivors are risk for increased stool frequency, incontinence, radiation proctitis, and perianal irritation, especially those treated with pelvic radiation.[31] Referral to a gastroenterologist or rectal surgeon should be considered if local steroid cream or foam is not effective.
- Uterine cancer survivors who have undergone radiation therapy may develop bladder and bowel dysfunction as well as atrophic vaginitis, sexual issues, and vaginal stenosis[32] (discussed previously).

PREVENTIVE CARE

The main focus in preventive care is on the prevention and detection of primacy cancer recurrence or second primary cancer (SPC) occurrence as well as providing other preventive services available to the general population.

- Primary care physician were found to be providing less counselling to cancer survivors compared to adults without cancer in three important areas of health behaviors: diet, exercise and smoking.[33]
- Screening for cervical cancer, cholesterol, and flu vaccination are also lower compared with the general population.[34]
- The MD Anderson Cancer Center and several other organizations have published algorithms for best practices in care delivery to cancer survivors.[35] The MD Anderson algorithms are standardized across all type cancers. The 4 key domains are (1) monitoring the primary cancer, (2) cancer prevention and early screening, (3) managing side effects from treatment, and (4) caring for the psychosocial functions.

- Four lifestyle and behavior changes can be targeted for preventive care: smoking cessation, maintaining a healthy weight, increasing physical activity, and improving nutrition.

Smoking Cessation

- In 2015, adult smoking rates among cancer survivors were 12.9% for men and 11.% for women.[36]
- The failure rate at first attempt is approximately 60% to 65%. Of those who quit, fewer than 25% remain smoke-free after a year.[37]
- Cancer survivors should be offered an intensive intervention that includes both behavioral as well as pharmacologic therapy. Meta-analyses in the 2008 Update, "Treating Tobacco Use and Dependence," demonstrated that abstinence rates improved with increasing number of therapy sessions and duration of treatment.
- Pharmacologic therapy included nicotine replacement therapy, bupropion-sustained release (SR), and varenicline. Drug combinations improve smoking cessation rates. Bupropion-SR and nicotine lozenge was superior to either of the drugs administered separately. A combination of nicotine patch and lozenge was the second-best therapy.[38] Varenicline combined with bupropion-SR has also been used to increase efficacy.[39] Adding bupropion-SR to varenicline may prevent developing depression and neuropsychiatric symptoms.[40]

Obesity

- Prevention of obesity should be a goal for all cancer survivors.
- In 2015, the estimated prevalence of obesity among survivors was 31.4%.[41] Having an ideal body weight may reduce the risk of developing cancers associated with obesity, such as colorectal, breast (in postmenopausal women) uterine, esophageal, renal, and pancreatic cancer.

Physical Activity

- Increasing physical activity is associated with improved quality of life and physical functioning in cancer survivors.
- A systematic review by Speck and colleagues[42] proved the beneficial effects of physical activity during or after active cancer treatment. Benefits include better self-esteem, less anxiety, and improved functional capacity and improvement in their general physical activity, aerobic fitness, and upper/lower body strength.
- Ballard-Barbash and colleagues[43] found cancers survivors who increased their physical activity after treatment had lower breast cancer recurrence and breast cancer–related death.
- American Cancer Society has recommended at least 150 minutes of moderate to vigorous intensity physical activity and 2 days of strength training on a weekly basis for cancer survivors.[44]

Comorbid Diseases

- Screening and treating for comorbid diseases is essential to improve survivorship.
- Age is also a risk factor for chronic diseases, such as diabetes, hypertension, coronary artery disease, and chronic obstructive pulmonary disease.
- Cancer survivors with diabetes compared with those without the disease were found to have 40% higher all-cause mortality rate.[45]

Nutrition

- The American Institute for Cancer Research/World Cancer Research Fund[46] and the American Cancer Society have published guidelines for nutrition and physical activity for cancer survivors.[44]
- A cancer-fighting diet is one based on increasing plant-based and decreasing animal-based food (meat, fish, poultry, and eggs).
- Simple advice for patients is to fill two-thirds of their plate with plant-based food (vegetables, fruits, whole grains, and legumes) and the remainder one-third with animal source food. Plant food contains antioxidants, such as β-carotene; lycopene; and vitamins A, C, and E, which are known to have a protective effect against free radicals. The phytochemicals in plants also can counteract the negative effect of carcinogens on cells.
- Red meat and processed meat consumption (smoked: A process of flavoring, browning, cooking, or preserving food by exposing it to smoke usually burning or smoldering material, most often wood. Cured: A process of preserving food by using combinations of salt, nitrates, nitrites, sugar and preservatives) have been associated with colorectal cancers.[46] N-nitroso compounds and heterocyclic amines (HCAs) and polycyclic aromatic hydrocarbons in processed meat foods are potent carcinogens. HCAs are produced from the smoke produced by the dripping of meat juices over fire, and the production of HCAs can be increased with certain cooking techniques (high temperature above 400° F, prolonged cooking time, frying, grilling, and char-boiling). Meat marinated with rosemary, mint, oregano, and sage reduces HCA during grilling due to content of polyphenolic antioxidants (carnosic acid, carnosol, and rosmarinic acid).
- Recommendations by the American Institute for Cancer Research is to limit red meat to no more than approximately 500gm per week.[47]

Consumption of Other Specific Items

- Sodium: intake should be under 2.4 g/d because the presence of salt in food increases N-nitroso compound formation.
- Alcohol: particularly when combined with smoking, alcohol is associated with head and neck cancer as well as with esophageal, breast, colorectal, and liver cancers. Limit to 1 drink per day if unable to abstain.
- Organic food: no evidence organic foods provide any cancer-protecting benefits.
- Vegetarian diet: may lower the risk of certain types of cancer (nasopharynx, mouth, pharynx, larynx, lung, pancreas, esophagus, stomach, colon, and rectum) but may lead to macronutrient or micronutrient deficiencies (eg, vitamin B_{12}, zinc, iron, and calcium) if it is not a balanced diet.
- Soy-based foods and breast cancer: a cohort study reported consumption of greater than or equal to 10 mg of soy isoflavones was associated with a statistically nonsignificant reduction in mortality but a statistically significant reduction in cancer recurrence.[48]
- There is high consensus for supplementing women who has breast and ovary cancer with vitamin D at a minimum daily dose of 800 IU. To attain the recommended serum target of 30 ng/ml and above may require prescribing 50,000 IU weekly for 8 weeks and then 800-1000 IU as a maintenance dose. Recommended dose for calcium is 1000 mg for women 19-50 years and 1200 mg for those 51-70 years.

Vaccination

- Cancer survivors are more susceptible to suffer from a vaccine-preventable disease and need to be current on their immunizations.

- In general, inactivated vaccines should be given 2 weeks before the start of chemotherapy or other immunosuppressive therapy. There is no harm in giving inactivated vaccines, but a full benefit is not attainable.[49]
- Attenuated live vaccines should be given 4 weeks prior to immunosuppressive therapy. The recommendation from the Infectious Diseases Society of America is to wait 3 months after immunosuppression therapy discontinuation to do it. For patients who are receiving anti–B-cell antibody, a 6-month wait is prudent.[50]
- Practical vaccination recommendations are provided in the study by Ariza-Heredia and colleagues.[51]

Fertility and Contraception

- PCHPs should explore cancer survivor patients' plans for family planning. PCHPs need to have the knowledge on indications and contraindications in the methods available for preserving fertility and in the use of contraception. Although the topic on family is too broad to cover in this article, salient points are mentioned to help referring patients to an appropriate specialist.
- Options of preserving fertility include embryo cryopreservation, cryopreservation of unfertilized oocytes, ovarian transposition (if pelvic radiation is done), ovarian tissue cryopreservation–future transplantation, and conservative gynecologic surgery. A detailed information can be reviewed in the clinical practice guideline.[52]
- Estrogen-containing or progesterone-containing contraceptives are contraindicated in hormonally mediated cancers, such as breast, endometrial, or those that have estrogen receptors (ERs) or progesterone receptors (PRs). Even when breast cancers are estrogen/progesterone-negative, use of hormonal contraception is contraindicated for the first 5 years [53]
- Use of copper (nonhormonal) intrauterine device is effective for contraception and does not have any related contraindications for breast cancer patients.
- A good reference to review safety of contraception for women with certain medical conditions is the US Medical Eligibility Criteria for Contraceptive Use, available at the Centers for Disease Control and Prevention Web site.[53]

RISK FOR FAMILY MEMBERS
Genetic Predisposition

- Only 5% to 10% of cancers are related to genetics. Approximately 50 hereditary cancer syndromes are linked to genetic changes or mutations. It is recommended that a geneticist be consulted before genetic screening is ordered. The criteria listed in **Box 1** can be used as guidelines for considering genetic testing of immediate family members.

Box 1
Criteria for considering genetic testing of immediate family members

Cancer diagnosed at an age that is unusual from the rest of the general population

Several different cancers occurring independently

Cancer occurring in both of any paired organs (eg, breast and kidney)

Several blood relatives having same kind of cancer (eg, mother, daughter, and sisters having breast cancer)

Unusual types of cancer (eg, breast cancer in a male relative)

Member of racial/ethnic group that is known to have an increased chance of having a certain hereditary cancer syndrome (eg, Ashkenazi Jews)

- Some of the hereditary cancers for which genetic testing is available are mentioned in the National Cancer Institute Web site[54] and are briefly elaborated.

Hereditary Breast and Ovarian Cancer Syndrome: Mutations in Genes BRCA1 and BRCA2

- Carriers of gene mutation have a high risk of breast and ovarian cancer. Mutations in the BRCA1 and BRCA2 genes may be suspected if breast cancer is diagnosed before age 50 or develops bilaterally or if there is simultaneous breast and ovarian cancer in either the same woman or within the same family, multiple breast cancers in family, or 2 or more primary types of BRCA1-related or BRCA2-related cancers in a single family member and from Ashkenazi Jewish ethnicity.

PTEN Hamartoma Tumor Syndrome: Gene PTEN

- PTEN mutation carriers have risk of cancer in several different organs. Highest to lowest cancer rates observed are for breast, thyroid, uterine, kidney, colorectal, and melanoma. Patients have small, noncancerous growths or hamartomas of the skin, mucous membranes, intestinal tract, or the brain. Family members can be tested for PTEN gene mutation.

Hereditary Non-polyposis (HNPN) Colorectal Cancer or Lynch Syndrome: Mutations of Genes MSH2, MLH1, MSH6, and PMS2

- Patients with genomic changes in mismatch repair genes are at high risk for early age colorectal and endometrial cancer. HNPN has been linked to mutations of MSH2, MLH1, MSH6 and PMS2. In addition, mutation of EPCAM has also been linked to several other organ specific cancers such as endometrium, ovary, breast, pelvic, pancreatic, small intestine, hepato-biliary tract, stomach and brain.

PROGNOSIS AND SURVIVAL
Recurrence

- Cancer recurrence can be either local (in the same place it first started), regional (in surrounding lymph nodes), or distant (in a different organ [eg, lungs, liver, bone, or brain]).
- Thorough history and physical examination remain the best options for detecting recurrence for breast cancer.
- Any new complaints require in-depth probing and a thorough physical examination. Local recurrence is usually detected by comprehensive examination of breast, chest wall, and lymph nodes.
- Distant metastasis should be highly suspected if they have concerning neurologic, pulmonary, and gastrointestinal symptoms. Unusual and persistent chest, abdominal, pelvic, or bone pain should raise concerns.
- Mammogram of breast is the only imaging method that can detect recurrence and is widely used in surveillance. There is no current evidence supporting that the use of breast MRI.

New Cancer

- Although a majority of SPCs (83%) are located in a new site, 13.2% occur in the same tissue as the first primary cancer and 2.3% occur in neighboring tissues.[55]

- Women are at higher risk than men for SPC in breast and gynecologic organs coupled with their gender-specific higher survival rates. The highest risk of SPC is noted when the first primary cancer is diagnosed at an early age (0–17 year old) and the lowest is among women who are 80 years or older.[56]
- There is no evidence-based algorithm to screen for SPC. PCHPs need to remain vigilant to be able to detect early occurrence based on knowledge of the 2 carcinogenic pathways, as outlined by Kreuger and colleagues.[57]

Lifestyle, Behavioral, or Environmental Risk factors

- Tobacco, alcohol, obesity, sun exposure, human papillomavirus (HPV), hepatitis B and hepatitis C, HIV, and *Helicobacter pylori* infection can be linked to SPC. Individuals with an HPV-related primary cancer seem to have a higher risk for genital, anal, or oral cancer.[58]

Treatment-Related Effects of Radiation Therapy and Chemotherapy

Ionizing radiation

Women who have undergone radiation to the chest for Hodgkin lymphoma have 3 times greater risk for developing breast or lung cancers.[59] The National Comprehensive Cancer Network Hodgkin lymphoma guidelines panel recommends initiating annual breast screening 8 years to 10 years post–chest or axilla radiation or at age 40 years, whichever comes first. In addition to mammogram, those who received radiation at ages 10 years to 30 years should also have MRI.[60]

Chemotherapy

Leukemia is the most common SPC associated among patients who have undergone prior chemotherapy treatment, in particular myelogenous leukemia and myelodysplasia syndrome.

SURVIVAL RATE

- When discussing survival, it is important to understand the terms used by oncologists and cancer researchers to provide straightforward answers.
- The term, *prognosis*, is used to refer to the likelihood of a desired outcome. Factors that can affect the prognosis of cancer are age, health status, stage at diagnosis, tumor grade, cell trait, treatment, and response to treatment.
- The term, *survival*, is defined as the time a person diagnosed with a disease is expected to live. Several statistics are used to predict survival for cancer patients. Relative survival is most commonly used to compare survival of people who have been diagnosed and/or treated for cancer compared with those who have not, over a certain period of time (usually a 5-year period), after controlling for age, gender, and race.
- A large proportion of female cancer survivors are those who were diagnosed with breast or other gynecologic malignancies. In 2016, mortality rates from those 2 types of cancer were 29% compared with 26% for lung and bronchial cancers. The survival rates of breast and gynecologic cancers are elaborated.

Breast Cancer (Adenocarcinoma)

- Factors that can affect breast cancer survival rate (**Table 1**) are tumor grade and ER, PR, and human epidermal growth factor receptor (HER2) status. Those with positive hormone receptors have better survival rates when drugs are used to block the receptors. Patients with a positive HER2 (protein marker) have breast cancer types that are more aggressive. Notwithstanding, there are drugs that

Table 1				
Breast cancer 5-year survival rates				
Cancer Stage	**I**	**II**	**III**	**IV**
5-y survival rate	95%	93%	72%	22%

kill the cells that produce HER2, thus improving survival. Triple-negative breast cancers (ER-negative, PR-negative and HER2-negative) have the lowest survival rates. Recent marker K167 have also been used to assess survival.

- The median age at diagnosis of breast cancer is 61 years.[61] With the advent of increased breast cancer screening, more than 61% of breast cancer cases in women are now diagnosed at a localized stage, with a favorable survival rate of 99% at 5 years. Overall relative survival rates for breast cancer at 5 years, 10 years, and 15 years are 89%, 83% and 78%, respectively.
- The National Cancer Institute has published breast cancer assessment tools,[62] based on Gail and colleagues' model,[63] to estimate a woman's chance of developing invasive breast cancer.
- Genomic Health[64] has launched genomic testing to provide a score for reoccurrence in newly diagnosed and early-stage breast cancers. Initially it was recommended for cases with ER-positive, HER2-negative, and node-negative.[65] Genomic test results help select the most appropriate therapy (hormonal or chemotherapy) and predict the probability of recurrence in distant sites. A unified consensus for health care providers to routinely use the test is lacking.
- A tool to predict outcome for ductal carcinoma in situ recurrence after breast conserving surgery has been developed and validated[66] and is available at a Web site hosted by Memorial Sloan Kettering Cancer Center.[67]

Uterine Cancer

- The median age at diagnosis of uterine cancer is 62 years.
- The 5-year and 10-year relative survival rates for women with uterine cancer are 82% and 79%, respectively (**Table 2** has further data on 5-year survival rates).
- A majority of uterine cancers (67%) are diagnosed at an early stage because of postmenopausal bleeding. Their 5-year survival rate is 95%. Overall, the 5-year survival rate is higher for whites (84%) than for African American women (62%).[56]
- A Web-based tool, hosted by the Memorial Sloan Kettering Cancer Center, using the International Federation of Gynecology and Obstetrics (Fédération Internationale de Gynécologie et d'Obstétrique) (FIGO) staging, grading system, and information on histopathology, is available to calculate survival after surgery.[68] Abu-Rustum and colleagues[69] published information on the nomogram used as a prediction tool.

Cervical Cancer

- Approximately 50% of cervical cancers are diagnosed at stage I with a 5-year survival rate of 90% (**Table 3** have further data on 5-year survival rates). After therapy, 35% have active cancer or a recurrence. In 2 years to 3 years, the rate of recurrence is 75%.

Table 2			
Uterine cancer 5-year survival rates			
Spread	**Localized**	**Regional**	**Distant**
5-y survival rate	95%	69%	17%

Table 3
Cervical cancer 5-year survival rates

Spread	Local Invasive	Surrounding Tissue and or Lymph Nodes	Distant Metastasis
5- year survival rate	91%	57%	17%

- Relapse depends on stage, histologic type (eg, small cell cancer has poor prognosis), tumor volume, depth of stromal invasion, and lymph–vascular space invasion. Relapse also depends on parametrical extension and lymph node involvement during the initial surgery and on surgeons' ability to get a cancer-free margin.[70]

Ovarian Cancer

Ovarian cancers are classified depending on the type of cell that it originated from. Survival depends on the type of ovarian cancer and the stage when diagnosed. (**Table 4** have further data according to type and stage).

Epithelial: About 90% of ovarian cancers develop in the epithelium. in early-stage ovarian cancer, the risk of relapse ranges from 15% to 40% or over, depending on staging and tumor grading (G1 and G2 have a better prognosis). For advanced stages, the overall recurrence rate is 80% after 2 years of treatment.

Stromal: Two most common types are granulosa cell tumors and sertoli-leydig cell tumors. Unlike the epithelial cancers, stromal cancers are diagnosed earlier. They rarely recur (only 10% of the time). Later recurrence, after 10 years denotes that the cancer is incurable.

Germ cell: Three most common types are teratomas, dysgerminomas and endodermal sinus tumors usually diagnosed at an early stage: stage I teratoma and dysgerminoma can be only treated surgically, with a 25% to 50% recurrence in abdomen and lymph nodes within 1 year to 2 years after treatment. Recurrence occurs in 1 year to 2 years.[71]

Table 4
Cancer stage and type 5-year survival rates

Stage	I	II	III	IV
Ovarian stromal	95%	78%	65%	35%
Ovarian germ cell	98%	94%	87%	69%
Fallopian tumor	87%	86%	52%	40%
Ovarian epithelial invasive	90%	70%	39%	17%

- A clinical tool to predict 5-year survival status post-surgery is available on the Web site hosted by the Memorial Sloan Kettering Cancer Center.[72] Known risk factors are history of hereditary breast and ovarian cancer syndrome, residual after debulking, histology, physical health of survivor, albumin level, and the FIGO tumor stage. Barlin and colleagues[73] created a nomogram that also can be used as clinical tool.

REFERENCES

1. Hoekstra RA, Heins MJ, Korevaar JC. Health care needs of cancer survivors in general practice: a systematic review. BMC Fam Pract 2014;15:94.

2. Rodriguez AR, FZ. Models of survivorship care. In: Aub MD, RSFM, editors. Advances in cancer survivorship management. New York: Springer; 2015.
3. Miller KD, Siegel RL, Lin CC, et al. Cancer treatment and survivorship statistics, 2016. CA Cancer J Clin 2016;66(4):271–89.
4. ABIM Foundation. Society of general internal medicine. Available at: http://www.choosingwisely.org/clinician-lists/society-general-internal-medicine-cancer-screening-in-adults-with-life-expectancy-less-than-10-years/. Accessed May 8, 2018.
5. Institute of Medicine (US) Committee on Psychosocial Services to Cancer Patients/Families in a Community Setting; Adler NE, Page AEK, editors. Cancer Care for the Whole Patient: Meeting Psychosocial Health Needs. Washington (DC): National Academies Press (US); 2008. Available at: https://www.ncbi.nlm.nih.gov/books/NBK4015/ doi: 10.17226/11993.
6. Dawes AJ, Hemmelgarn M, Nguyen DK, et al. Are primary care providers prepared to care for survivors of breast cancer in the safety net? Cancer 2015; 121(8):1249–56.
7. Society AC. Cancer treatment and survivorship. Facts and figures 2016-2017. Atlanta (GA): American Cancer Society; 2016.
8. Cohen EE, LaMonte SJ, Erb NL, et al. American Cancer Society head and neck cancer survivorship care guideline. CA Cancer J Clin 2016;66(3):203–39.
9. American Cancer Society. Guidelines for the early detection of cancer. Available at: https://www.cancer.org/healthy/find-cancer-early/cancer-screening-guidelines/american-cancer-society-guidelines-for-the-early-detection-of-cancer.html. Accessed May 8, 2018.
10. Pachman DR, Barton DL, Swetz KM, et al. Troublesome symptoms in cancer survivors: fatigue, insomnia, neuropathy, and pain. J Clin Oncol 2012;30(30): 3687–96.
11. Cramp F, Byron-Daniel J. Exercise for the management of cancer-related fatigue in adults. Cochrane Database Syst Rev 2012;11:CD006145.
12. Epstein DR, Dirksen SR. Randomized trial of a cognitive-behavioral intervention for insomnia in breast cancer survivors. Oncol Nurs Forum 2007;34(5):E51–9.
13. Mustian KM, Sprod LK, Janelsins M, et al. Multicenter, randomized controlled trial of yoga for sleep quality among cancer survivors. J Clin Oncol 2013;31(26): 3233–41.
14. van den Beuken-van Everdingen MH, de Rijke JM, Kessels AG, et al. Prevalence of pain in patients with cancer: a systematic review of the past 40 years. Ann Oncol 2007;18(9):1437–49.
15. Levy MH, Chwistek M, Mehta RS. Management of chronic pain in cancer survivors. Cancer J 2008;14(6):401–9.
16. Fausti S. Audiologic monitoring for ototoxicity and patient management 230-251. Pharmacology and ototoxicity for audiologist. In: Campbell KCM, editor. Clifton Park (NY): Thomson/Delmar Learning; 2006.
17. Brawley O, Byers T, Chen A, et al. New American Cancer Society process for creating trustworthy cancer screening guidelines. JAMA 2011;306(22):2495–9.
18. Mitchell AJ, Ferguson DW, Gill J, et al. Depression and anxiety in long-term cancer survivors compared with spouses and healthy controls: a systematic review and meta-analysis. Lancet Oncol 2013;14(8):721–32.
19. Barbera L, Zwaal C, Elterman D, et al. Interventions to address sexual problems in people with cancer. Curr Oncol 2017;24(3):192–200.
20. Mead H, Cartwright-Smith L, Jones K, et al. Racial and ethnic disparities in US health care. A chartbook. New York: The Commonwealth Fund; 2008.

21. de Moor JS, Virgo KS, Li C, et al. Access to cancer care and general medical care services among cancer survivors in the United States: an analysis of 2011 medical expenditure panel survey data. Public Health Rep 2016;131(6):783–90.

22. DiSipio T, Rye S, Newman B, et al. Incidence of unilateral arm lymphoedema after breast cancer: a systematic review and meta-analysis. Lancet Oncol 2013;14(6): 500–15.

23. Kummerow KL, Du L, Penson DF, et al. Nationwide trends in mastectomy for early-stage breast cancer. JAMA Surg 2015;150(1):9–16.

24. Gamelin E, Gamelin L, Bossi L, et al. Clinical aspects and molecular basis of oxaliplatin neurotoxicity: current management and development of preventive measures. Semin Oncol 2002;29(5 Suppl 15):21–33.

25. Lehky TJ, Leonard GD, Wilson RH, et al. Oxaliplatin-induced neurotoxicity: acute hyperexcitability and chronic neuropathy. Muscle Nerve 2004;29(3):387–92.

26. Durand JP, Deplanque G, Montheil V, et al. Efficacy of venlafaxine for the prevention and relief of oxaliplatin-induced acute neurotoxicity: results of EFFOX, a randomized, double-blind, placebo-controlled phase III trial. Ann Oncol 2012;23(1): 200–5.

27. Loprinzi CL, Reeves BN, Dakhil SR, et al. Natural history of paclitaxel-associated acute pain syndrome: prospective cohort study NCCTG N08C1. J Clin Oncol 2011;29(11):1472–8.

28. Hitchcock YJ, Tward JD, Szabo A, et al. Relative contributions of radiation and cisplatin-based chemotherapy to sensorineural hearing loss in head-and-neck cancer patients. Int J Radiat Oncol Biol Phys 2009;73(3):779–88.

29. Theunissen EA, Zuur CL, Bosma SC, et al. Long-term hearing loss after chemo-radiation in patients with head and neck cancer. Laryngoscope 2014;124(12): 2720–5.

30. Tell R, Lundell G, Nilsson B, et al. Long-term incidence of hypothyroidism after radiotherapy in patients with head-and-neck cancer. Int J Radiat Oncol Biol Phys 2004;60(2):395–400.

31. Lange MM, Martz JE, Ramdeen B, et al. Long-term results of rectal cancer surgery with a systematical operative approach. Ann Surg Oncol 2013;20(6): 1806–15.

32. Tada H, Teramukai S, Fukushima M, et al. Risk factors for lower limb lymphedema after lymph node dissection in patients with ovarian and uterine carcinoma. BMC Cancer 2009;9:47.

33. Sabatino SA, Coates RJ, Uhler RJ, et al. Provider counseling about health behaviors among cancer survivors in the United States. J Clin Oncol 2007 May 20; 25(15):2100–6.

34. Earle CC, Neville BA. Under use of necessary care among cancer survivors. Cancer 2004;101(8):1712–9.

35. MD Anderson Cancer Center. Cancer survivorship algorithm. Available at: https://www.mdanderson.org/for-physicians/clinical-tools-resources/clinical-practice-algorithms/survivorship-algorithms.html. Accessed October 17, 2017.

36. National Cancer Institute. Cancer trends progress report: cancer survivors and smoking. Available at: https://progressreport.cancer.gov/after/smoking.

37. Treating tobacco use and dependence 2008 update. Clinical Practice Guideline; 2008. Available at: https://www.ncbi.nlm.nih.gov/books/NBK63952.

38. Smith SS, McCarthy DE, Japuntich SJ, et al. Comparative effectiveness of 5 smoking cessation pharmacotherapies in primary care clinics. Arch Intern Med 2009;169(22):2148–55.

39. Ebbert JO, Croghan IT, Sood A, et al. Varenicline and bupropion sustained-release combination therapy for smoking cessation. Nicotine Tob Res 2009; 11(3):234–9.

40. Karam-Hage M, Shah KR, Cinciripini PM. Addition of bupropion SR to varenicline alleviated depression and suicidal ideation: a case report. Prim Care Companion J Clin Psychiatry 2010;12(2) [pii:PCC.09l00800].

41. National Cancer Institute. Cancer trend progress report: cancer survivors and obesity. 2017. Available at: https://progressreport.cancer.gov/after/obesity.

42. Speck RM, Courneya KS, Mâsse LC, et al. An update of controlled physical activity trials in cancer survivors: a systematic review and meta-analysis. J Cancer Surviv 2010;4(2):87–100.

43. Ballard-Barbash R, Friedenreich CM, Courneya KS, et al. Physical activity, biomarkers, and disease outcomes in cancer survivors: a systematic review. J Natl Cancer Inst 2012;104(11):815–40.

44. Rock CL, Doyle C, Demark-Wahnefried W, et al. Nutrition and physical activity guidelines for cancer survivors. CA Cancer J Clin 2012;62(4):243–74.

45. Barone BB, Yeh HC, Snyder CF, et al. Long-term all-cause mortality in cancer patients with preexisting diabetes mellitus: a systematic review and meta-analysis. JAMA 2008;300(23):2754–64.

46. World Cancer Research Fund/American Institute for Cancer research. Food, nutrition, physcial activity and the prevention of cancer: a global perspective second expert report. Washington, DC: 2007.

47. Smith JS, Ameri F, Gadgil P. Effect of marinades on the formation of heterocyclic amines in grilled beef steaks. J Food Sci 2008;73(6):T100–5.

48. Nechuta SJ, Caan BJ, Chen WY, et al. Soy food intake after diagnosis of breast cancer and survival: an in-depth analysis of combined evidence from cohort studies of US and Chinese women. Am J Clin Nutr 2012;96(1):123–32.

49. Rubin LG, Levin MJ, Ljungman P, et al. 2013 IDSA clinical practice guideline for vaccination of the immunocompromised host. Clin Infect Dis 2014;58(3):309–18.

50. Berglund A, Willén L, Grödeberg L, et al. The response to vaccination against influenza A(H1N1) 2009, seasonal influenza and Streptococcus pneumoniae in adult outpatients with ongoing treatment for cancer with and without rituximab. Acta Oncol 2014;53(9):1212–20.

51. Ariza-Heredia EJ, Chemaly RF. Practical review of immunizations in adult patients with cancer. Hum Vaccin Immunother 2015;11(11):2606–14.

52. Oktay K, Harvey BE, Partridge AH, et al. Fertility preservation in patients with cancer: ASCO clinical practice guideline update. J Clin Oncol 2018;36(19): 1994–2001.

53. CDC. Summary chart of Medial Eligibility Criteria (MEC) for contraceptive Use. 2017. Available at: https://www.cdc.gov/reproductivehealth/contraception/pdf/summary-chart-us-medical-eligibility-criteria_508tagged.pdf. Accessed February 5, 2018.

54. National Cancer Institute. Genetic testing fact sheet. Genetic testing for hereditary cancer syndromes. Available at: https://www.cancer.gov/about-cancer/causes-prevention/genetics/genetic-testing-fact-sheet. Accessed October 2017.

55. Fraumeni J, Curtis R, Edwards BEA. New malignancies among cancer survivors: SEER cancer registries 1973-2000. Bethesda (MD): NCI; 2006.

56. SEER cancer statistic review. (CSR) 1975-2014; 2017.

57. Krueger H, McLean D, Williams D. The prevention of second primary cancers. Progress in experimental tumour research, vol. 40. New York: Karger AG Basel; 2008.

58. Hisada M, Rabkin S. Viral causes of cancer. In: Shields PG, editor. Cancer risk assessment. Boca Raton (FL): Taylor & Francis; 2005.

59. Travis LB, Gospodarowicz M, Curtis RE, et al. Lung cancer following chemotherapy and radiotherapy for Hodgkin's disease. J Natl Cancer Inst 2002;94(3): 182–92.

60. network Ncc. Hodgkin lumphoma. 2018. Accessed April 24, 2018.

61. Siegel RL, Miller KD, Jemal A. Cancer statistics, 2016. CA Cancer J Clin 2016; 66(1):7–30.

62. Breast cancer assessment tool. Available at: https://www.cancer.gov/bcrisktool/.

63. Gail MH, Brinton LA, Byar DP, et al. Projecting individualized probabilities of developing breast cancer for white females who are being examined annually. J Natl Cancer Inst 1989;81(24):1879–86.

64. Oncotype DX. Available at: https://online.genomichealth.com/Login.aspx.

65. American Society of Clinical Oncology. Use of biomarkers to guide decisions on adjuvant systemic therapy for women with early-stage invasive breast cancer. 2016. Available at: https://www.asco.org/practice-guidelines/quality-guidelines/ guidelines/breast-cancer -/9746. Accessed October 16, 2017.

66. Rudloff U, Jacks LM, Goldberg JI, et al. Nomogram for predicting the risk of local recurrence after breast-conserving surgery for ductal carcinoma in situ. J Clin Oncol 2010;28(23):3762–9.

67. Tool to predict ductal carcinoma in situ. Available at: http://nomograms.mskcc. org/breast/DuctalCarcinomaInSituRecurrencePage.aspx.

68. Tool for survival probability after surgery for uterine cancer. Available at: https:// www.mskcc.org/nomograms/endometrial/post_op.

69. Abu-Rustum NR, Zhou Q, Gomez JD, et al. A nomogram for predicting overall survival of women with endometrial cancer following primary therapy: toward improving individualized cancer care. Gynecol Oncol 2010;116(3):399–403.

70. Salani R, Backes FJ, Fung MF, et al. Posttreatment surveillance and diagnosis of recurrence in women with gynecologic malignancies: Society of Gynecologic Oncologists recommendations. Am J Obstet Gynecol 2011;204(6):466–78.

71. Colombo N, Carinelli S, Colombo A, et al. Cervical cancer: ESMO clinical practice guidelines for diagnosis, treatment and follow-up. Ann Oncol 2012;23(Suppl 7): vii27–32.

72. Memorial Sloan Kettering Cancer Center. Tool to predict predict the likelihood of surviving epithelial ovarian cancer for five years after surgery. Available at: https://www.mskcc.org/nomograms/ovarian/post_op.

73. Barlin JN, Yu C, Hill EK, et al. Nomogram for predicting 5-year disease-specific mortality after primary surgery for epithelial ovarian cancer. Gynecol Oncol 2012;125(1):25–30.

Women's Health and the Military

Carissa van den Berk Clark, PhD, MSW[a], Jennifer Chang, MD[b],
Jessica Servey, MD[c], Jeffrey D. Quinlan, MD[b],*

KEYWORDS

- Veteran • Military sexual trauma • Intimate partner violence • PTSD

KEY POINTS

- Women in the military face unique reproductive health risks during and after completion of service, including infertility, increased risk of hysterectomy, and sexually transmitted illness.
- Among active duty women, the rate of unintended pregnancy is approximately 60% and is associated with low utilization rates of long-acting reversible contraceptives.
- Intimate partner violence and military sexual assault are important risk factors for developing posttraumatic stress disorder (PTSD). Active duty women and female veterans should be screened for both.
- Female veterans experience more potentially traumatic events than civilian women. PTSD is a primary mechanism linking these events to poor health among female veterans.
- Women veterans are at higher risk of cardiovascular disease, obesity, gastrointestinal disorders, and chronic pain than their civilian counterparts.

INTRODUCTION

Approximately 1.8 million American women are veterans of the Armed Services (representing 9.4% of all veterans), and this number is expected to increase by approximately 18,000 women per year for the next 10 years.[1] In addition, more than 200,000 women (14.6% of the total force) are currently serving on active duty.[1] With the increasing number of women in the military, there has been a similar increase in the number of women who have faced prolonged deployment in combat environments and who have had support roles in combat. In addition to the physical and behavioral health issues covered in the rest of this issue, these women may have considerations

Disclosure Statement: The authors have nothing to disclose.
[a] Department of Family and Community Medicine, School of Medicine, Saint Louis University, 1402 South Grand Boulevard, St Louis, MO 63104, USA; [b] Department of Family Medicine, F. Edward Hebert School of Medicine, Uniformed Services University of the Health Sciences, 4301 Jones Bridge Road, Bethesda, MD 20814, USA; [c] Department of Family Medicine, Faculty Development, F. Edward Hebert School of Medicine, Uniformed Services University of the Health Sciences, 4301 Jones Bridge Road, Bethesda, MD 20814, USA
* Corresponding author.
E-mail address: jeffrey.quinlan@usuhs.edu

specific to their service in the armed forces. In particular, this article discusses reproductive health concerns, family planning and contraceptive considerations, intimate partner violence (IPV) and military sexual assault, posttraumatic stress disorder (PTSD), and postdeployment health issues. It concludes with a list of available resources accessible to veterans and their providers.

ASSESSING FOR VETERAN STATUS

Given the number of women who are either serving on active duty or who have served on active duty, it is important for physicians to identify this important demographic in women for whom they provide care. Patients may not readily volunteer this information, and therefore, providers should incorporate questioning about military service into their standard demographics data collection. Asking if the patient currently serves or has ever served in the military will provide an introduction to further questioning. In patients who have served, it is important to determine how long they served and if they are eligible for either TRICARE (military and retiree health insurance) or Veterans Health Administration (VHA) benefits. Assessment for health risk should include determining if they have served overseas, on a ship, and/or in combat or other austere environments. In addition, patients should be asked about potential harmful exposures, history of IPV, military sexual trauma (MST), and history of behavior health concerns, including specifically, PTSD.

REPRODUCTIVE HEALTH CONCERNS

Women in the military face unique reproductive health risks during and after completion of service. Limited access to bathrooms in deployed settings has been associated with poor vaginal hygiene and increased rates of vaginitis.[2] Postponed urination and intentional fluid restriction in the deployed setting are associated with urinary retention and urinary tract infection. These physiologic and hygiene challenges may predispose to development of chronic urogenital problems, especially in women suffering from comorbid mental health conditions. Overactive bladder affects 22% of women veterans, twice the rate in the general population, and may be related to these deployment challenges as well as to lifetime sexual trauma, PTSD, and depression.[2] Although rates of stress urinary incontinence and pelvic organ prolapse are unknown, it is likely that delayed voiding during deployments and strenuous military jobs, such as paratrooper training, increase the risks.[2]

For most servicewomen, a large percentage of their time on active duty is spent during the childbearing years. Sixteen percent of female veterans who have served in the Iraq and Afghanistan conflicts report a lifetime history of infertility.[2] Although it is unknown if the causes of infertility among veterans are related to unique occupational exposures within the military, research has demonstrated that infertility among servicewomen is associated with a history of lifetime sexual assault.[2] The Department of Veterans Affairs provides basic infertility evaluation, surgical procedures, and some interventions, such as intrauterine insemination, and medications to induce ovulation for veterans with infertility. In vitro fertilization is not covered except for in cases involving combat-related urogenital injury.[2]

Women veterans have an increased risk of hysterectomy during the premenopausal period; the mean age of those undergoing hysterectomy is 35, significantly lower than in the civilian sector.[3] This risk of hysterectomy is further potentiated by a history of completed sexual assault (with vaginal penetration) and a history of PTSD. This risk is also related to an increase in gynecologic symptoms, including pelvic pain, abnormal bleeding, and pelvic inflammatory disease.[3]

Women veterans are at increased risk for certain sexually transmitted infections (STIs) and have higher levels of lifetime sexual activity, including younger age at first intercourse and higher number of partners, than nonveterans. Although higher rates of herpes simplex virus-2 positivity and self-reported genital warts are seen in women veterans, less is known about the risk of chlamydia compared with nonveterans.[4] Comprehensive health care for women veterans should include age- and risk-appropriate screenings for cervical cancer and other STIs.

FAMILY PLANNING AND CONTRACEPTIVE CONSIDERATIONS

Among active duty women, the rate of unintended pregnancy is approximately 60%, but the rate is unknown among women veterans, owing in large part to the fact that many veterans seek care outside of the VHA.[5] Demographic risks of unintended pregnancy include younger age, unmarried status, lower socioeconomic levels, and lower military rank. In addition, among women veterans, unintended pregnancy is associated with racial and ethnic minority status and with IPV.[5] Both lack of contraceptive use and use of less effective contraceptive methods contribute to unintended pregnancy among active duty women.[5] Surveys have shown that 60% of active duty women with unintended pregnancy were not using contraception at the time of conception.[5] In response, there is a growing body of efforts that targets both service member education and increasing provider knowledge and competency in contraceptive options, including long-acting reversible contraceptives (LARC), described in later discussion.

Among active duty women, there are lower rates of the more effective LARC methods, such as intrauterine device (IUD) and implant, as compared with oral contraceptives; however, rates of LARC usage are improving.[5] Barriers to effective contraceptive use in the deployed setting are listed in **Table 1**. Emergency contraception (EC) may reduce unplanned pregnancy for active duty women. Barriers to use of EC include ethical concerns by the patient or lack of patient or provider knowledge in prescribing EC.[5] Both TRICARE and the VHA cover EC for women who request it.

Table 1
Barriers to contraceptive use in the deployed setting

Type of Barrier	Specific Examples
Side effects of medication	Headaches Nausea Weight gain Irregular bleeding patterns
Environmental hazards affecting adherence	Oral contraceptives • Changing time zones • Long shifts/hours • Changing work schedules Patch • Difficulty with adhesion in hot environments and wear of heavy gear Multiple methods (pill, patch, ring) • Limited storage • Privacy concerns
Access to care	Limited options on formulary Difficulty obtaining refills Lack of provider knowledge or skill Limited provider options (including gender)

Data from Goyal V, Borrero S, Schwarz EB. Unintended pregnancy and contraception among active-duty servicewomen and veterans. Am J Obstet Gynecol 2012;206(6):463–9.

Health care for women veterans of reproductive age should include inquiry into reproductive goals and need for contraception. Unintended pregnancy may pose significant threats to women veterans and their fetuses, especially among those at risk for homelessness, PTSD, depression, and chronic medical conditions.[2] Up to 50% of women veterans of child-bearing age may receive prescriptions for potentially teratogenic medications, and up to 60% may not receive counseling on contraception before starting new medications.[6] Women veterans reporting a history of MST are more likely to receive contraceptive services and to use women's health clinics as compared with those without a history of MST.[7]

Contraceptive services within the Veterans Administration (VA) system include provision of a 3-month supply of medication, limited co-pay requirements, complete coverage for IUDs and their insertion, streamlined processes for obtaining refills, and EC.[5] Access to LARC for women veterans varies by location and availability of providers skilled in comprehensive women's health. Rates of LARC usage among women veterans who are or have ever been homeless are approaching the rates in the general population, particularly among those from more recent Iraq and Afghanistan conflicts.[6] Although access to contraception seems to be increasing for women veterans, further improvements are needed.

Active duty servicewomen have limited access to abortion; per Department of Defense legislation, abortion is prohibited except when the life of the mother is endangered if the pregnancy were carried to term or when a pregnancy is the result of rape or incest.[2] Access to abortion and abortion counseling are currently prohibited by the Department of Veterans Affairs.[2]

INTIMATE PARTNER VIOLENCE AND MILITARY SEXUAL TRAUMA

IPV includes stalking, physical assault, and rape by an intimate partner. In the civilian population, 29% of women experience IPV during their lifetimes.[8] Although the data are heterogeneous in nature, the VHA reports that women veterans have a slightly increased rate of 35%.[9] IPV is important for both the acute trauma that it causes and the potential for long-term consequences. These long-term consequences include several adverse health outcomes and behaviors, including the development of chronic pain, PTSD and other behavioral health diagnoses, and substance abuse, such as tobacco and alcohol use disorders.[10] Ultimately, poorer health in victims of IPV leads to increased health care utilization in women who have experienced it.[10]

Care for these patients often requires a multidisciplinary approach. Acute physical injuries should be cared for appropriately and behavioral health concerns addressed using evidence-based approaches, such as cognitive behavioral therapies. In addition, these patients may require significant social support, such as legal services, education and employment assistance, housing and childcare, and assistance meeting other financial needs.[10]

MST refers to either threatening sexual harassment or sexual assault that occurs during military service. It includes incidents of quid pro quo, in which women are pressured to engage in sexual activity in order to seek favorable action or avoid negative action as well as sexual interactions that they were unable to consent to, such as while intoxicated. Risk factors for MST are multifactorial but likely include the dynamics of deployment, military culture itself, and the perception and/or reality that offenders face little to no punishment for their actions.

It is difficult to fully assess the incidence of MST because there are several reasons that victims may not report the incident or seek care; however, one meta-analysis found that 38.4% of female service members and veterans reported a history of

MST.[11] Potentially even more concerning is that 12% of women in one study reported MST having occurred during deployment.[12] Female veterans also have a high lifetime prevalence of sexual assault (38%–64%).[13] As a result of the prevalence of MST, both the Department of Defense and the VA have mandated routine screening for all patients. Screening includes 2 questions: "While you were in the military, (1) did you receive uninvited and unwanted sexual attention, such as touching, cornering, pressure for sexual favors, or verbal remarks? (2) Did someone ever use force or threat of force to have sexual contact with you against your will?"[14]

A variety of evidence-based cognitive behavioral therapies have been shown to be effective for the treatment of MST. These therapies include prolonged exposure therapy, interpersonal therapy, cognitive processing therapy, and eye movement desensitization reprocessing therapy.[15] Women who have experienced MST are eligible for care at no cost from the VHA for the treatment of medical conditions related to their trauma. In patients identified as having been a victim of MST who are not currently receiving care at the VHA, consideration should be given to referring them to the nearest facility for care. Information on how to refer is found at the end of this article.

POSTTRAUMATIC STRESS DISORDER

Several studies have shown that PTSD is a primary mechanism linking potentially traumatic events (PTE) to poor health among female veterans.[13] Most female veterans screening positive for PTSD and depression also have unmet medical health needs (59%), and they often identify affordability as a reason for delaying care.[16] Given the known effect of combat exposure and PTSD on health outcomes, the VHA has led the way in the United States in the delivery of integrated health care with universal screenings of PTSD, MST, body mass index, and pain.[17]

Female veterans experience higher rates of PTEs than civilian females, between 81% and 93% compared with 51.2% and 68.9%.[18] As shown in **Table 2**, a large proportion of female veterans see combat[19] even if they did not serve in direct combat roles. As mentioned previously, they experience high rates of IPV and MST. Furthermore, female veterans face substantially higher interpersonal stressors than male veterans,[19] problems fitting in,[16] separation from children and family, and poor social support.[20]

Several studies have shown that female veterans experience similar rates of PTSD as their male counterparts and higher levels of depression.[21] Although men are more

Table 2	
Rates of potentially traumatic exposure and psychiatric disorders among female veterans	
Item	**Percentage, %**
Trauma (all)	81–93
Trauma (combat)	4–73.4
Trauma (MST)	25–50
PTSD	21–23
TBI	11
Depression	48
Alcohol misuse	4–37
Binge drinking	7–25
Chronic pain	5

Abbreviation: TBI, traumatic brain injury.

likely to experience trauma in their lifetimes, women are much more likely to develop PTSD.[18] Several studies have shown gender differences in trauma response patterns.[22] Although men are more likely to develop more sensitive hyperarousal systems (symptoms related to impulse control, aggression, and hypervigilance), women are more likely to develop more sensitized dissociative systems (symptoms related to anxiety, withdrawal, depression). Women's coping styles also are more emotive and avoidance focused (ie, disengagement, social isolation, self-destructive behaviors) than men.[22]

Women also are more prone to problematic substance use and use substances differently than men.[22,23] The differences have attributed to environmental context, that is, women's environmental systems may be more likely to influence substance use/dependence because they lack personal resources and social power. In addition, because relationships are often a priority to women, they may use substances as a way to bond with their partner and maintain the relationship. Meanwhile, such use increases the likelihood of abuse and violence and further decreases the likelihood of behavioral health utilization by increasing stigma and dependence on partners.[23] On the whole, studies have mostly found relationships among central nervous depressants (alcohol, heroine, and so forth) and patients experiencing hyperarousal symptoms. Studies show that the central nervous system stimulant cocaine is more commonly used by patients experiencing emotional distress.[23]

Box 1 provides recommendations for treating female veterans with a focus on mental health wellness. Given that only about 40% of female veterans are currently using the VHA, many civilian doctors will be caring for this population. Providing quality care for female veterans means using many of the evidence-based practices that have been incorporated by the VHA for military/veteran populations. These practices include consistent screeners, integrated care, trauma-informed practices, cognitive behavioral treatments for PTSD and substance use treatments like motivational interviewing, intensive outpatient treatment, family counseling and medications for alcohol, smoking, and opioid dependence.

Box 1
Recommendations for treating female veterans

- Civilian providers should consistently use VA screeners for PTSD, MST, and pain for female veterans
- Have mental health resources available so that coordination of care is smooth
- Use of Screening, Brief Intervention, and Referral to Treatment to screen for alcohol use and to facilitate motivation to quit or cut down
- Be prepared to educate female veterans about their rights to access VA services
- Focus heavily on depression and depression care because almost half of female veterans suffer from depression
- Family therapy and relationship counseling should be considered during stages of deployment
- Loss of appetite and appraisal of distress are higher among women with PTSD than men; physicians should determine how distress is affecting health choices, such as healthy eating and substance use
- Offer telemedicine/Web approaches (85% have Web access)[2]
- Sexual assault survivors are sensitive to touch; given the high prevalence of MST and sexual assault among female veterans, ask before you touch female veterans

POSTDEPLOYMENT HEALTH RISKS

Women veterans have multiple health risks outside of mental health disorders, and the vast array of gynecologic issues, including contraceptive concerns and sexual assault consequences discussed above. The next section expands the current known information of women veterans' risk of cardiovascular disease, obesity, gastrointestinal disorders, and chronic pain.

Even though cardiovascular disease is the leading cause of death in women, women tend to develop this approximately a decade later than men. Direct comparisons of cardiovascular risk between women veterans versus those who have never served in the military have not been done. However, women veterans are developing cardiovascular risk factors at a higher rate. It is thought that these increased rates of individual risk factors may affect early cardiovascular disease. Studies from the Department of Veterans Affairs demonstrate that approximately one-fourth of women veterans already have more than 2 cardiovascular risk factors by the time they are between 45 and 54, and between 55 and 64 that increases to one-third of women veterans.[24] For hypertension specifically, women veterans have a 28% 10-year incidence of hypertension compared with a 13% 10-year incidence for civilians.[25] Although these comparisons are not exact, they represent the closest age and time comparisons available. In a large study of women veterans who, by self-report, were physically inactive or had current mental health symptoms (depressive, anxiety, or PTSD), their risk for cardiovascular disease was statistically increased.[26] Furthermore, PTSD is an independent risk factor for the development of cardiovascular disease in women veterans.[27] Other research has demonstrated a larger percent of women veterans who smoke compared with men. In a large study of 65,627 people, 29% of women veterans smokes versus 23% of men, and were younger. Furthermore, despite being counseled to quit more often than men, women veterans have a lower smoking cessation rate.[28] The increased risk of this combination of cardiovascular risk contributes to higher overall cardiovascular risk.

Even though obesity is only one of many cardiac risk factors, it has surpassed the others in notable risk for women veterans. Forty-four percent of women veterans are obese.[29] In a study on new cardiac risk factor diagnoses, the only one cardiac risk factor that women were more likely to develop than men was obesity.[25] Further analysis demonstrated statistical differences in rates of obesity exist between those women with depression (hazard ratio [HR] = 1.17) versus those without depression (HR = 1.01).[25] Obesity is a multifactorial disease that also has subsequent health risks, such as diabetes and hyperlipidemia. It may be that the research has not yet demonstrated increased rates of these other risk factors pending longer studies. Early data suggest that women veterans may prefer gender-specific clinics for their medical care.[26] Further research is needed to develop the best plan for caring for women veterans and the biggest impact to change their development of cardiovascular disease and specifically obesity.

Functional gastrointestinal disorders are more common in women than men in the general population. In women veterans, both irritable bowel syndrome (IBS) and dyspepsia potentially occur in higher rates than civilian comparisons.[30] In a study of women veterans, having concomitant depression, anxiety, or PTSD increased the odds of reporting symptoms of IBS and dyspepsia.[30] Having unwanted sexual contact also increased their risk of these functional disorders.[31]

Finally, chronic pain occurs often in women veterans. Chronic pain has been noted as the number of women veterans, especially those who have experienced deployments, have increased over the past 15 years. Studies have suggested increased rates of mastalgia, menstrual disorders, and chronic pelvic pain; this risk may increase further if the patient has PTSD or past sexual trauma.[32] Compared with male veterans, women are more likely to develop chronic musculoskeletal pain, and this may be related to differences in injury rates.[33] In a large study of men and women veterans, women had a higher rate of multiple musculoskeletal pain disorders than men, 19.4% versus 15.7%.[34] Women are more likely to report moderate to severe pain on rating scales than men.[34] These findings may lead to increased disability or increased pain medication. Research has yet to delineate these more functional findings. Women veterans may need more proactive screening regarding musculoskeletal pain and dysfunction, and treatment plans mindful of the need to avoid opioid overuse.

REFERRALS/RESOURCES

As indicated in the text of this article, women veterans who are suffering from any of these issues or other service-related illnesses are eligible to seek care in the VHA. Patients and providers can obtain further information on local resources by using the Web-based facility directory (www.va.gov/directory) or by calling the VHA at 1-800-827-1000. In addition, for patients with PTSD or providers caring for patients with PTSD, there are several additional resources available. These resources include the National PTSD Information Hotline, which can be e-mailed at ncptsd@va.gov or can be reached by telephone at 1-802-296-6300. Educational resources are available for providers through the National Center for PTSD (http://www.ptsd.va.gov/professional/ptsd101/ptsd-101.asp). Finally, several mobile applications are available for the public (https://www.ptsd.va.gov/public/materials/apps/PTSDCoach.asp) and providers (https://www.ptsd.va.gov/professional/materials/apps/index.asp) through the VA.

REFERENCES

1. Statistics National Center for Veterans Analysis and Statistics. Women veterans report: the past, present and future of women veterans. Washington, DC: Department of Veteran Affairs; 2017.
2. Zephyrin LC. Reproductive health management for the care of women veterans. Obstet Gynecol 2016;127(2):383–92.
3. Ryan GL, Mengeling MA, Summers KM, et al. Hysterectomy risk in premenopausal-aged military veterans: associations with sexual assault and gynecologic symptoms. Am J Obstet Gynecol 2016;214(3):352.e1-13.
4. Lehavot K, Katon JG, Williams EC, et al. Sexual behaviors and sexually transmitted infections in a nationally representative sample of women veterans and nonveterans. J Womens Health (Larchmt) 2014;23:246–52.
5. Goyal V, Borrero S, Schwarz EB. Unintended pregnancy and contraception among active-duty servicewomen and veterans. Am J Obstet Gynecol 2012; 206(6):463–9.
6. Gawron LM, Redd A, Suo Y, et al. Long-acting reversible contraception among homeless women Veterans with chronic health conditions: a retrospective cohort study. Med Care 2017;55:S111–20.
7. Goyal V, Mattocks K, Schwarz EB, et al. Contraceptive provision in the VA Healthcare System to women who report military sexual trauma. J Womens Health 2014; 23(9):740–5.
8. Black MC, Basile KC, Breiding MI. National intimate partner and sexual violence survey: 2010 summary report. Atlanta (GA): Center of Disease Control and Prevention; 2011.

9. Gierisch JM, Shapiro A, Grant NN, et al. Intimate partner violence: prevelance among US military veterans and active duty service members and review of intervention approaches. Washington, DC: Department of Veteran Affairs; 2013.

10. Gerber MR, Iverson KM, Dichter ME, et al. Women veterans and intimate partner violence: current state of knowledge and future directions. J Womens Health 2014;23(4):302–9.

11. Wilson LC. The prevalence of military sexual trauma: a meta-analysis. Trauma Violence Abuse 2016. 1524838016683459.

12. Burns B, Grindlay K, Holt K, et al. Military sexual trauma among US servicewomen during deployment: a qualitative study. Am J Public Health 2014; 104(2):345–9.

13. Zinzow HM, Grubaugh AL, Monnier J, et al. Trauma among female veterans: a critical review. Trauma Violence Abuse 2007;8(4):384–400.

14. Kimerling R, Gima K, Smith MW, et al. The Veterans Health Administration and military sexual trauma. Am J Public Health 2007;97(12):2160–6.

15. Valente S, Wight C. Military sexual trauma: Violence and sexual abuse. Military Medicine 2007;172(3):259–65.

16. Lehavot K, Der-Martirosian C, Simpson TL, et al. Barriers to care for women veterans with posttraumatic stress disorder and depressive symptoms. Psychol Serv 2013;10(2):203–12.

17. Haskell SG, Mattocks K, Goulet JL, et al. The burden of illness in the first year home: do male and female VA users differ in health conditions and healthcare utilization. Womens Health Issues 2011;21(1):92–7.

18. Suffoletta-Maierle S, Grubaugh AL, Magruder K, et al. Trauma-related mental health needs and service utilization among female veterans. J Psychiatr Pract 2003;9(5):367–75.

19. Street AE, Gradus JL, Giasson HL, et al. Gender differences among veterans deployed in support of the wars in Afghanistan and Iraq. J Gen Intern Med 2013; 28(Suppl 2):S556–62.

20. Street AE, Vogt D, Dutra L. A new generation of women veterans: stressors faced by women deployed to Iraq and Afghanistan. Clin Psychol Rev 2009;29(8):685–94.

21. Fulton JJ, Calhoun PS, Wagner HR, et al. The prevalence of posttraumatic stress disorder in Operation Enduring Freedom/Operation Iraqi Freedom (OEF/OIF) Veterans: a meta-analysis. J Anxiety Disord 2015;31:98–107.

22. Olff M, Langeland W, Draijer N, et al. Gender differences in posttraumatic stress disorder. Psychol Bull 2007;133(2):183.

23. Najavits LM, Weiss RD, Shaw SR. The link between substance abuse and posttraumatic stress disorder in women. A research review. Am J Addict 1997;6(4): 273–83.

24. Vimalananda VG, Miller DR, Christiansen CL, et al. Cardiovascular disease risk factors among women veterans at VA medical facilities. J Gen Intern Med 2013;28(2):517–23.

25. Haskell SG, Brandt C, Burg M, et al. Incident cardiovascular risk factors among men and women veterans after return from deployment. Med Care 2017;55(11):948–55.

26. Goldstein KM, Oddone EZ, Bastian LA, et al. Characteristics and health care preferences associated with cardiovascular disease risk among women veterans. Womens Health Issues 2017;27(6):700–6.

27. Ahmadi N, Hajsadeghi F, Mirshkarlo HB, et al. Post-traumatic stress disorder, coronary atherosclerosis, and mortality. Am J Cardiol 2011;108(1):29–33.

28. Farmer M, Rose D, Riopelle D, et al. Gender differences in smoking and smoking cessation treatment: an examination of the organizational features related to care. Womens Health Issues 2011;21(4S):S182–9.
29. Breland JY, Phibbs CS, Hoggatt KJ, et al. The obesity epidemic in the Veterans Health Administration: Prevalence among key populations of women and men Veterans. J Gen Intern Med 2017;32(1):11–7.
30. Savas LS, White DL, Wieman M, et al. Irritable bowel syndrome and dyspepsia among women veterans: prevalence and association with psychological distress. Aliment Pharmacol Ther 2009;29(1):115–25.
31. White DL, Savas LS, Daci K, et al. Trauma history and risk of the irritable bowel syndrome in women veterans. Aliment Pharmacol Ther 2010;32(4):551–61.
32. Levander X, Overland M. Care of women veterans. Med Clin North Am 2015;99: 651–62.
33. Haskell SG, Gordon KS, Mattocks K, et al. Gender differences in rates of depression, PTSD, pain, obesity, and military sexual trauma among Connecticut War Veterans of Iraq and Afghanistan. J Womens Health (Larchmt) 2010;19(2):267–71.
34. Higgins DM, Fenton BT, Driscoll MA, et al. Gender differences in demographic and clinical correlates among veterans with musculoskeletal disorders. Womens Health Issues 2017;27(4):463–70.

Best Practices in Transgender Health
A Clinician's Guide

Jessica Lapinski, DO[a],*, Tiffany Covas, MD, MPH[b],
Jennifer M. Perkins, MD, MBA[c], Kristen Russell, MSW, LCSW[d],
Deanna Adkins, MD[e], Melanie Camejo Coffigny, JD[f],
Sharon Hull, MD, MPH[g]

KEYWORDS

- Transgender health • LGBTQ health • Organ inventory • Gender affirming care
- Annual examination • Transgender mental health

KEY POINTS

- Transgender patients often look for subtle clues in the office environment to suggest that the practice is transgender friendly; as such, creating a trans-affirming practice is a crucial first step to providing competent care.
- Providers should perform an annual organ inventory and keep this up to date in their electronic medical record system to help guide preventative screenings.
- As a general rule, if an individual has a particular body part or organ and otherwise meets criteria for screening based on risk factors or symptoms, screening should proceed, regardless of hormone use.
- There are standard guidelines for initiation and continuation of hormone replacement therapy; however, it is important to have an open dialogue with your patient regarding their goals of therapy and reasonable expectations.

Disclosure Statement: The authors have nothing to disclose.
[a] Department of Community and Family Medicine, Duke University Health System, Duke University, 2100 Erwin Road, Durham, NC 27710, USA; [b] Department of Community and Family Medicine, Duke University Health System, 2100 Erwin Road, Durham, NC 27710, USA; [c] Division of Diabetes, Endocrinology, and Metabolism, Department of Medicine, Duke University Health System, 2100 Erwin Road, Durham, NC 27710, USA; [d] Department of Case Management, Duke Child and Adolescent Gender Care, Duke University Health System, 2100 Erwin Road, Durham, NC 27710, USA; [e] Duke Child and Adolescent Gender Care, Duke University Health System, 2100 Erwin Road, Durham, NC 27710, USA; [f] Duke University, 2100 Erwin Road, Durham, NC 27710, USA; [g] Department of Community and Family Medicine, Duke University School of Medicine, 2100 Erwin Road, Durham, NC 27710, USA
* Corresponding author.
E-mail address: jessica.lapinski@duke.edu

Prim Care Clin Office Pract 45 (2018) 687–703
https://doi.org/10.1016/j.pop.2018.07.007
0095-4543/18/© 2018 Elsevier Inc. All rights reserved.
primarycare.theclinics.com

INTRODUCTION

Providing culturally competent and medically knowledgeable care to the transgender and the gender nonconforming community is increasingly requested and falls within the realm of primary care practice. This patient population has unique health care needs, is subject to a variety of health care disparities, and is often reticent to seek medical care owing to prior negative experiences.[1] Few medical schools, medical residency programs, or training programs for advanced practice providers provide formal training in this arena.[2] The purpose of this article is to offer current primary care clinicians an overview of best practices as they relate to health care for transgender individuals. This article is by no means a comprehensive guide, but is intended as a starting point for clinicians so that they may provide high-quality, affirming, and value-based care to their transgender patients.

HEALTH DISPARITIES AND SOCIAL DETERMINANTS OF HEALTH

Social determinants of health often contribute to health disparities among vulnerable populations. In the transgender population, relevant social determinants include chronic stress, higher rates of homelessness, unemployment, frequent victimization, and high Adverse Childhood Events scores.[3] One study suggested that 28% of transgender individuals were harassed in medical settings, 19% were denied care, and 2% experienced violence.[4] Owing to inconsistent access to health care in general, and more specifically gender-affirming care, the transgender population is at increased risk of experiencing retraumatization in medical settings.[5] Approximately one-fifth of the transgender population has experienced homelessness, 12% of whom have been homeless within the last year.[6] Income disparities exist with poverty levels twice the nation average and a high rate of people in the lowest income bracket (<$10,000 per year).[4] Of those who were out (had disclosed their gender identity and/or sexual orientation) to their immediate family, 10% reported experiencing violence and 8% were kicked out of the house because of their disclosure.[6]

Relevant medical literature supports the premise that the intersection between being a gender minority (ie, transgender) and a racial minority is associated with increased rates of poverty, unemployment, and greater health disparities when compared with the Caucasian transgender population.[6] Disabled and undocumented people who are transgender experience increased discrimination as well.[3] Environmental factors that affect the health of lesbian, gay, bisexual, transgender (LGBT) individuals include legal discrimination, a lack of laws protecting children from bullying in schools, a lack of social programs, and a shortage of health care providers who are knowledgeable and culturally competent.[3]

Other factors that contribute to this population's health disparity include high uninsured rates and greater reliance on public insurance.[6] For example, only 40% of transgender individuals had access to employer health insurance compared with 62% of cisgender individuals (one whose gender identity matches their sex assigned at birth).[6] Another source of disparities in LGBT health care comes from a long history of anti-LGBT bias in health care that has resulted in fewer people from this population seeking care and to an overall decrease in access to care.[7] Access to knowledgeable providers willing to care for transgender patients is limited. Homophobia and transphobia persist in some health care settings, with limited emphasis during training on cultural empathy or understanding among health care professionals, which presents challenges for the provision of appropriate primary care.[8–11] Additionally, challenges for aging or disabled patients include finding skilled nursing facilities, rehabilitation units, and/or assisted living facilities that allow rooming in for same sex couples, allow family of choice to make medical decisions, set appropriate visitation parameters, and respect the gender identity of transgender patients.[12] **Table 1** includes selected key health disparities in the transgender population.

CREATING A TRANS-AFFIRMING PRACTICE

Research suggests that LGBT patients often search for subtle cues in the environment to determine if a practice is friendly.[13] Because of this, it is crucial for practices to create a gender-affirming environment throughout the clinical practice. Characteristics of such an environment are varied and impact all aspects of the practice. Intake forms should be inclusive of a wide range of gender identities and patients should be addressed by their preferred pronoun(s).[13] All staff should be trained to refer to patients by their preferred pronouns and their correct gender identity. The physical office space should display LGBT-friendly symbols, stickers, photographs, and posters representing a diverse patient population.[13] Brochures in the waiting room should include material pertinent to the transgender community. Within the examination room, the clinician should foster a welcoming environment by asking open, nonjudgmental questions. The provider should ask about the patient's gender identity and their preferred pronoun(s), which should be used when addressing the patient throughout the visit.[13] The provider should feel confident in conducting an organ inventory (described elsewhere in this article), which should guide preventive care for the patient. Ideally, the electronic health record (EHR) should be able to capture sexual orientation and gender identity information accurately for purposes of patient care and appropriate handling of insurance and billing functions.[14–16]

THE ELECTRONIC HEALTH RECORD

The EHR can become a barrier to care for transgender patients if it does not incorporate appropriate collection of sexual orientation and gender identity data.[15] Key components of appropriate sexual orientation and gender identity data collection include capture of the patient's preferred name, gender at birth, sexual orientation, and gender identity.[14–16] If the EHR is not built to collect these data appropriately at registration and intake, many difficulties can arise for the patient and the provider entity. Problems can include nonaffirming experiences for patients called by the wrong name, identified by inappropriate pronouns, or treated incorrectly based on provider or staff assumptions about sex, gender identity, and sexual orientation and behaviors. Surgeries appropriate to the patient's situation may be denied or questioned based on incorrect assumptions about gender identity or the presence or absence of organs. Laboratory tests that are appropriate for the patient's gender identity may be reported with the incorrect reference ranges based on gender as reported in the EHR. Patients may also be denied insurance payment for appropriate health care services and provider entities may encounter significant billing and compliance issues because of inaccurate data used in health care documentation.

UNDERSTANDING THE MEANING OF "TRANSITIONING" FOR TRANSGENDER PATIENTS

The process of transitioning one's gender is complex and varies from individual to individual.[17] Individuals may complete some, none, or all of the components of the 3 broad categories of transitioning (social, medical, and surgical) over the course of their lifetimes.[17] Underlying the decision to transition requires identification of the dysphoria brought about through identification with the sex and gender roles assigned at birth

Table 1
Key health disparities in the transgender population

	Key Transgender Health Disparities
Youth[6,47–51]	• LGBT youth are 2–3 times as likely to attempt suicide • LGBT youth are more likely to be homeless • Homeless youth who are LGBT are more likely to report victimization, substance abuse, and to have more sexual partners and more psychopathology than their heterosexual comparison • Youth are frequently bullied at school and are more likely to be victims of sexual violence than their peers according the Youth Risk Behavior Survey in 2016 • At school (K-12) youth who were perceived as transgender were likely to be verbally harassed (54%), physically attacked (24%), and sexually assaulted (13%), resulting in 17% of kids leaving school owing to the environment • HIV prevalence in male-to-female youth varied from 19% to 22%, showing them to be at high risk for infection
Access[3,6]	• Transgender individuals are less likely to have health insurance than heterosexual or LGB counterparts • 29% of the transgender population lives in poverty compared with 12% of the US population • One-third of USTS respondents had a negative experience with a health care provider related to being transgender within the last year • 23% of USTS participants did not seek health care owing to fear of being mistreated • 25% of USTS participants had a health insurance problem related to being transgender in the last year • 55% of USTS participants had sought coverage for surgery and were denied • 25% of USTS participants had sought care for hormones and were denied • 33% of USTS participants did not go to a health care provider owing to the expense • The unemployment rate in the transgender population in the USTS survey was 15% compared with 5% in the cisgender population

Infections[51–53]	• Some studies suggest a disparity in the availability of HIV treatment services. A recent four-city study found that transgender women were less likely to receive highly active antiretroviral therapy than a control group of MSM, heterosexual women and men, and male intravenous drug users
	• Hepatitis C prevalence rates between 11% and 24% and hepatitis B rates from 4% to 76% among specific samples of transgender women are estimates based on limited studies
	• A prevalence rate of tuberculosis of up to 13% among transgender women in San Francisco
	• HIV infection is highest among transgender women of color, with HIV prevalence rates ranging from
	  ○ 41% to 63% among African-American transgender women
	  ○ 4% to 50% among Latina transgender women
	  ○ 4% to 13% among Asian-Pacific Islander transgender women
	• HIV prevalence in transgender men (female to males) is estimated to range from 2% to 3%, which is still elevated compared with cisgender men
	• Some limited research has found elevated rates of sexually transmitted diseases with varying prevalence rates of
	  ○ Syphilis (3%–79%)
	  ○ Gonorrhea (4%–14%)
	  ○ Chlamydia (2%–8%)
	  ○ Herpes (2%–6%)
	  ○ Human papillomavirus (3%–7%)

(continued on next page)

Table 1 (*continued*)	
Key Transgender Health Disparities	

Substance abuse[21,51,54]	• Adolescents are 2.5 to 5.0 times more likely to use substances (including vaping, smoking, drinking, heavy episodic drinking) than their nontransgender peers
	• Transgender adolescent youth are at higher risk of recent substance use and earlier onset of substances, which increases risk for long-term addiction
	• Increased gender and sexuality based harassment is associated with increased substance abuse at every grade
	• Some studies have shown that marijuana, crack cocaine, and alcohol are the most commonly used drugs by transgender people
	• Studies have also found alarming rates of methamphetamine use (4%–46%) and injection drug use (2%–40%)
	• Some studies suggest that tobacco use rates can range from 45% to 74%
	• Access to substance abuse treatment services can be very difficult for transgender people. Studies have suggested that barriers to treatment services often include:
	  ○ Discrimination,
	  ○ Provider hostility and insensitivity,
	  ○ Strict binary gender (male/female) segregation within programs, and
	  ○ Lack of acceptance in gender-appropriate recovery groups.

Obesity[50]	• LGBT youth have higher rates of obesity, which predisposes to metabolic syndrome and diabetes
Cancer[55–59]	• Transgender men were more likely to have an inadequate pap than cisgender women and this increased with duration of testosterone therapy • Transgender men were less likely to be up-to-date on pap screenings (AOR, 0.63; $P<.01$) • Although rare, there is an increased risk for vaginal, cervical, and endometrial cancer with hormone therapy • Male to female transgender persons are not at higher risk than biological women for breast cancer and thus not recommended for screening mammography • Association between masculinizing hormone therapies and elevated liver enzymes, loss of bone mineral density, and increased risk for ovarian cancer • Underutilization of health care in general and limited screening owing to gender mismatch
Mental health[6,48,60]	• 39% had serious psychological distress in the previous month compared with only 5% of the US population • Higher rates of depression and anxiety • When compared with MSM and bisexually active women, transgender women were most likely to report depressive symptoms and suicidal ideation
Suicide[6]	• 40% of respondents in the USTS had attempted suicide in their life time compared with 4.6% of the general population • 7% had attempted suicide in the last year compared with 0.6% in the US population
Violence[6,37]	• Approximately 66% of transgender people have been sexually assaulted in their lifetime • 50% of undocumented transgender individuals had been homeless in their lifetime and 68% had faced intimate partner violence • 16%–60% of transgender people are victims of physical assault or abuse • Social stigmatization and other factors may additionally lead to an underreporting of acts of violence committed against transgender people

Abbreviations: MSM, men who have sex with men; USTS, US transgender survey.

and acknowledgment of a desire to see oneself and to be seen by others as a different sex and/or gender. Throughout different components of transitioning, sexual orientation can change.[18] This fluctuation tends to occur more commonly with individuals who are attracted to the opposite biological sex before transitioning.

Social transition includes the decision to present publicly as one's gender identity and may include changes in appearance, use of pronouns, preferred name, and sexual behaviors and partnering.[17] Social/behavioral interventions include resocialization efforts to learn the mannerisms, communication, and interactions styles of the preferred gender, tucking of the penis or binding of the breasts, and voice coaching. Support for mental health conditions, screening for depression and anxiety, and assessment of readiness to begin medical transition is important in this phase of transition.

Medical, or endocrine, transition includes the decision to seek medical (typically hormonal) therapy to shift the appearance and function of hormone-producing organs, hair growth patterns, and other outward signs gender.[17] World Professional Association for Transgender Health has developed Standards of Care that include diagnosing gender dysphoria, treating comorbid conditions and making sure mental health conditions are stable, education about the medical treatment under consideration, and the ability to give consent before medical treatment.[19] Ideally, this phase of transition includes mental health support, including management of mood, anxiety, and other conditions. A systemic review of the effects of hormone therapy on psychological functioning showed a statistically significant improvement in mental health conditions during the transition and affirming process.[20]

Surgical transition includes the surgical augmentation of internal and external hormone and sex-related organs.[17] Options include surgery to remove the Adam's apple (tracheal shave), orchiectomy, vaginoplasty, and breast augmentation for male-to-female individuals. For female-to-male transitioning patients, surgical options include mastectomy, hysterectomy and salpingo-oophorectomy, metoidoplasty, phalloplasty, and sexual reassignment surgery.

THE HISTORY AND PHYSICAL EXAMINATION
General Considerations

When taking a patient's history and conducting a physical examination, it is crucial to do so in a gender-affirming way. History taking should be done in an open, nonjudgmental fashion, considering individualized changes and characteristics in the setting of hormone administration and/or surgical interventions that have taken place. The clinician should be sensitive to potential prior negative experiences and trauma, especially within the health care environment.[4] Physical examination should be relevant to the anatomy that is present, regardless of gender presentation. Providers should have an understanding that secondary sexual characteristics may present on a spectrum of development in patients transitioning with hormone therapy and somewhat depend on the durations of use and age at initiation.

The Organ Inventory

An organ inventory is an anatomic survey that allows providers to record the organs each patient has at any given point in time.[21] Such an inventory should be conducted annually for all transgender patients. Once someone has transitioned socially, medically, and/or surgically, they may change their gender marker in the medical record. It then becomes important to know sex assigned at birth, current hormone-producing organs, and current exogenous hormones. An organ inventory allows providers to maintain a record of the patient's medical transition history and current anatomy. In turn, this inventory drives routine health care screenings that a patient requires. A sample organ inventory is displayed in **Box 1**.

The Physical Examination

There are likely to be special considerations with regard to the pelvic examination in both male-to-female and female-to-male patients. In transgender females who have undergone gender reassignment surgery, the anatomy of the neovagina differs from a natal vagina.[21] It is a blind cuff, without a cervix or surrounding fornices and could have a more posterior orientation. Because of this, an anoscope should be used when visual inspection is necessary.[21] For the transgender male, the clinician should have an understanding that the pelvic examination may be traumatic or induce anxiety.[21] Transgender men are less likely to be up to date on cervical cancer screenings and have a higher rate of inadequate cytologic sampling.[21] Additionally, it is imperative to make clear to the laboratory that the sample provided is a cervical pap smear even, if the gender listed is male to avoid incorrect handling of the specimen.[21]

Other special considerations include chest binding and tucking of the testicles and penis. Chest binding is done to create a more masculine appearance of the chest; however, it may lead to skin breakdown or other complications of the skin.[22] Patients may be hesitant to remove the binder during an examination.[23] Safe binding education is recommended for all trans male patients who have not undergone mastectomy. Tucking of the testicles and penis may lead to hernias or other complications at the external inguinal ring or the potential for skin breakdown at the perineum.[22] Thorough

---

Box 1
Sample organ inventory

Organ inventory

Cervix

Uterus

Natal vagina

Neophallus

Penis

Prostate

Testes

Neovagina

Organ inventory with laterality

Left breast

Left fallopian tube

Left ovary

Left testis

Right breast

Right fallopian tube

Right ovary

Right testis

and sensitive history taking, examination, and education are recommended for all transgender patients.[22]

Hormonal Therapy: Consideration of Risks

When caring for transgender patients, the clinician should counsel on risks of cross-sex hormone therapy, particularly before the initiation of therapy and at each subsequent visit, weighing the risks and benefits to guide therapeutic decision making. It is critical to consider risks in the context of family history and medical comorbidities. Unsupervised hormone therapy is not advised[24] and physicians should ask patients about any history of previous hormone use not under the supervision of a medical provider.

For transgender females using estrogen therapy, high-risk adverse outcomes include thromboembolic disease, and moderate risk adverse outcomes includes hyperprolactinemia, breast cancer, coronary artery disease, cerebrovascular disease, cholelithiasis, and hypertriglyceridemia.[25] Given these risks, it is strongly recommended for clinicians to encourage tobacco cessation, although smoking is not an absolute contraindication to estrogen. If a transgender female has a prior history of a sex hormone–responsive cancer (breast or pituitary), consultation with an oncologist before initiating therapy is critical.[21] Antiandrogen therapy is typically used in prostate cancer therapy; however, there is less clear of a role of estrogen on the development of prostate cancer.[26] For those with family history or personal history of venous thromboembolism, an anticoagulative workup should take place to guide decision making in antiplatelet or anticoagulation therapy.[21] Routine prophylaxis with antiplatelet therapy is not recommended based on current evidence. In patients with a high risk of venous thromboembolism, the preferred route of administration of estrogen is transdermal to minimize risk because it avoids first-pass liver metabolism and induction of clotting factor production.[21] Although no evidence exists to strongly support the use of 81 mg/d aspirin in smokers, it can be considered as an additional preventive measure while using informed assessment of the risk versus benefit between venous thromboembolism prevention and gastrointestinal hemorrhage. As with cisgender women, avoidance of synthetic estrogens other than 17 beta estradiol and conjugated estrogens decreases the risk of venous thromboembolism by nearly one-half.[21]

In transgender males, the use of testosterone carries a very high risk of erythrocytosis (hematocrit >50%) and moderate risk of severe liver dysfunction (transaminases >3 times the upper limit of normal). The risk for coronary artery disease, cerebrovascular disease, and hypertension increases to that of a cisgender male. There may also be an increased risk for breast and/or uterine cancer.[25]

For both transgender males and females, it is important to avoid supraphysiologic dosing of sex steroids because the associated risks are more likely to arise and are worsened in this scenario.[27] The most recent Endocrine Society guidelines recommend regular clinical evaluation for physical changes and potential adverse outcomes after initiation of sex hormones and laboratory evaluation of sex steroids hormone levels every 3 months during the first year of therapy for both male and female transgender patients, then once or twice yearly.[25]

Monitoring of Hormonal Therapy

The endocrine transition provides an important opportunity for appropriate regular medical monitoring. Clinicians should monitor weight and blood pressure and conduct appropriate physical examinations. They should assess various health questions, including tobacco use, symptoms of depression, adverse effects of sex steroids, and symptoms concerning for deep vein thrombosis or pulmonary embolism.[28]

For transgender males, the goal of therapy is to maintain testosterone in the physiologic normal male range while avoiding adverse events resulting from excess testosterone therapy such as erythrocytosis, sleep apnea, hypertension, excessive weight gain, salt retention, lipid changes, and excessive or cystic acne.[29] In contrast with the Endocrine Society guidelines, the University of California San Francisco (UCSF) guidelines recommend against routine screening for lipids and hemoglobin A1c and recommend following the United States Preventative Services Task Force guidelines to drive decision making.[21] The UCSF guidelines also recognize that serum total testosterone has limitations owing to fluctuations in gonadotropins and recommend calculating the bioavailable testosterone using the total testosterone, albumin and sex hormone–binding globulin with a general reference range of greater than 72 ng/dL.[21] **Box 2** illustrates the current monitoring plan for transgender males as per the Endocrine Society guidelines[25] and **Table 2** provides the UCSF recommended guidelines.[21]

For transgender females either on estrogens, gonadotropin suppression, or antiandrogens, key issues include avoiding supraphysiologic doses or blood levels of estrogen that put the patient at a greater risk of thromboembolic disease, liver dysfunction, or elevations in blood pressure. Clinicians should choose a quality controlled assay for measuring serum estradiol levels to avoid measurement challenges.[30] In a study examining a large Dutch cohort, the risk of venous thromboembolism was shown to be 20-fold increased in Dutch transgender patients using estrogen.[31] This increase may have been associated with the use of the synthetic estrogen, ethinyl estradiol.[32] Given this finding, the use of synthetic estrogens and conjugated estrogens is not recommended because of the inability to monitor and dose based on serum levels in the setting of venous thromboembolism risk.[25] Additionally, in transgender females, periodic prolactin assessment is recommended by the Endocrine Society,[25] because estrogen therapy may increase the growth of pituitary lactotroph cells. Several reports

---

Box 2
Monitoring of transgender males on gender affirming hormone therapy as recommended by the Endocrine Society guidelines

- Clinical evaluation and monitoring every 3 months in the first year and then every 6 to 12 months appropriate signs of virilization and for development of adverse events.

- Measure serum testosterone every 3 months until levels are in the physiologic male range.
  - For intramuscular preparations, measure midway. The target is 400 to 700 ng/dL.
  - Transdermal testosterone can be measured following 1 week of daily application at least 2 hours after application.

- Measure hematocrit or hemoglobin at baseline and then every 3 months in the first year of therapy. Monitor weight, blood pressure, and lipids at regular intervals.

- Screening for osteoporosis should be undertaken in those who stop testosterone therapy, who develop risks for bone loss, or are nonadherent with therapy.

- If cervical tissue is present, regular screening as recommended by the American College of Obstetricians and Gynecologists.

- Ovariectomy can be considered after completion of hormone transition.

- Conduct annual breast examinations if mastectomy is performed and, if not, then consider mammograms as recommended by the American Cancer Society.

From Hembree WC, Cohen-Kettenis PT, Gooren L, et al. Endocrine treatment of gender-dysphoric/gender-incongruent persons: an Endocrine Society clinical practice guideline. J Clin Endocrinol Metab 2017;102(11):3890; with permission.

Table 2
Monitoring of therapy for transgender males: University of California San Francisco guidelines

Parameter	Baseline	Additional Monitoring
Lipids	No evidence supporting, use discretion. Monitor as per USPSTF guidelines	PRN
Hemoglobin A1C or fasting glucose	No evidence supporting, use discretion. Monitor as per USPSTF guidelines	PRN
Estradiol	Not indicated	PRN
Total testosterone	Not indicated	3, 6 and 12[a] months then PRN
Sex hormone-binding globulin[b]	Not indicated	3, 6 and 12[a] months then PRN
Albumin[b]	Not indicated	3, 6 and 12[a] months then PRN
Hematocrit and hemoglobin	Measure	3, 6, 12[a] months, yearly and PRN

Abbreviations: PRN, pro re nata (as needed); USPSTF, US Preventative Services Task Force.
  [a] In first year of therapy only.
  [b] Used to calculate bioavailable testosterone; monitoring bioavailable testosterone is optional and may be helpful in complex cases.
  Adapted from Deutsch MB. Guidelines for the primary and gender-affirming care of transgender and gender nonbinary people. 2nd edition. Available at: http://transhealth.ucsf.edu/pdf/Transgender-PGACG-6-17-16.pdf. Accessed November 12, 2017; with permission.

have demonstrated the development of prolactinomas occurring after long-term, high-dose estrogen therapy, and up to 20% of transgender females treated with estrogens may have elevations in prolactin levels.[33] In contrast, the UCSF guidelines recommend against routine prolactin screening unless there is evidence of visual disturbances, excessive galactorrhea, or new onset of headaches.[21] Last, in general, reference ranges for laboratory values used in monitoring hormonal therapy should take into consideration the identified gender, not the physiologic gender.[21] **Box 3** displays recommended monitoring in transgender females per the Endocrine Society[25] and **Table 3** per the UCSF guidelines.[21]

MENTAL HEALTH AND THE TRANSGENDER PATIENT

Current medical, psychological, and social research has increasingly shown that, while being transgender is not a mental disorder or medical condition, gender dysphoria, the manifestation of psychological distress brought on by the dissonance between assigned gender and felt gender, is a condition that can be treated.[34] The treatments discussed above are affirming of patients' gender identity and can help transgender youth and adults facilitate a successful gender transition. There is increasing evidence that this approach leads to improved health and mental health outcomes.[35–37] To be clear, the treatment of gender dysphoria does nothing to resolve the social stigma, discrimination, oppression, and health disparities that contribute to the high rates of unemployment (double the national average), harassment (78%), physical (61%) or sexual assault (64%), homelessness (double the national average), depression (35%–58%), anxiety (25%), eating disorders (7%), and suicide ideation (51%) and suicide attempts (41%) within the transgender population.[4,38–42] These concerns can be easily screened for during medical visits.

Box 3
Monitoring of transgender females on gender affirming hormone therapy as recommended by the Endocrine Society guidelines

- Evaluate patient every 3 months in the first year and then 6 to 12 months to monitor for appropriate signs of feminization and for development of adverse reactions.

- Measure serum testosterone and estradiol levels every 3 months.
  - Goal serum testosterone level is less than 50 ng/dL.
  - Serum estradiol should not exceed the peak physiologic range: 100 to 200 pg/mL.

- For patients taking spironolactone, serum electrolytes including potassium should be monitored every 3 months in the first year and annually thereafter.

- Routine cancer screening is recommended as in nontransgender individuals (all tissues present).

- Consider bone mineral density testing at baseline. In patients at low risk, screening for osteoporosis should be conducted at 60 years of age or in those who are not compliant with hormone therapy.

From Hembree WC, Cohen-Kettenis PT, Gooren L, et al. Endocrine treatment of gender-dysphoric/gender-incongruent persons: an Endocrine Society clinical practice guideline. J Clin Endocrinol Metab 2017;102(11):3890; with permission.

Transgender or gender diverse adolescents are especially vulnerable, because they are experiencing gender identity development at the same time that they may be exploring their sexual orientation, while also going through puberty and navigating high school. Coming out to friends and family, managing school policy around using

---

Table 3
Monitoring of therapy for transgender females: University of California San Francisco guidelines

Parameter	Baseline	Additional Monitoring
Lipids	No evidence supporting, use discretion. Monitor as per USPSTF guidelines.	PRN
A1C or fasting glucose	No evidence supporting, use discretion. Monitor as per USPSTF guidelines.	
Estradiol	Not indicated.	3, and 6[a] months, PRN
Total testosterone	Not indicated.	3, 6 and 12[a] months then PRN
Sex hormone–binding globulin[b]	Not indicated.	3, 6 and 12[a] months then PRN
Albumin[b]	Not indicated.	3, 6 and 12[a] months then PRN
Prolactin	Only if symptoms of prolactinoma.	PRN
Bun/Cr/K[c]	Measure.	3, 6, 12[a] months, yearly and PRN

Abbreviations: BUN/Cr/K, blood urea nitrogen, creatinine, potassium; PRN, pro re nata (as needed); USPSTF, US Preventative Services Task Force.
[a] In first year of therapy only.
[b] Used to calculate bioavailable testosterone; monitoring bioavailable testosterone is optional and may be helpful in complex cases.
[c] For patients on spironolactone only.
Adapted from Deutsch MB. Guidelines for the primary and gender-affirming care of transgender and gender nonbinary people. 2nd edition. Available at: http://transhealth.ucsf.edu/pdf/Transgender-PGACG-6-17-16.pdf. Accessed November 12, 2017; with permission.

the bathroom or locker room, and having preferred name and pronouns used appropriately by others are just a few experiences unique to transgender youth. The amount of psychosocial stress that is endured by these youth cannot be overstated. In just 1 clinic, the Transgender Health Clinic at Cincinnati Children's, 30% of the transgender youth that they served reported at least 1 suicide attempt; a history of self-injury was reported by 42% of the youth they served.[43]

Clinicians in a primary care setting are often in an optimal position to provide support to transgender individuals. Understanding the risks and recognizing that transgender patient's access to medical or mental health care may be limited is key in maximizing the work that can be done during their visit.

CONSIDERATIONS FOR SPECIAL POPULATIONS
Pediatric and Adolescent Patients

There is no universal treatment path that can, or should, be applied to all transgender children and youth. Often, treatment includes 1 or more of the following: psychotherapy, social transition, use of puberty blockers to delay the onset of puberty, hormone replacement therapy, and surgical options for young adults, 18 or older. All of these treatments can be used in an effort to relieve gender dysphoria by helping to align one's body with one's gender identity, allowing the individual to live and present in the world as the gender they authentically feel themselves to be.

In minor children presenting with gender dysphoria for a period of over 6 months who have not yet started puberty or who have not yet progressed beyond Tanner stage II of puberty, the suggested treatment includes supportive efforts to help the child explore their gender identity.[25] This process may include support from a mental health provider trained in working with gender diverse children, efforts toward social transition, and the possible use of puberty blockers (leuprolide or histrelin). Puberty blockers are medications that suppress the increase of testosterone and estrogen in the body, delaying puberty until the blockers are discontinued. Because puberty blockers have been used for decades in children with precocious puberty,[44] they are considered a safe alternative to having a child with gender dysphoria progress through a puberty that they feel is incorrect and therefore exacerbates gender dysphoria and increases the risk of self-harm, including suicide.[25] This treatment option buys the patient some time to continue gender identity development and exploration until they are older and can make a more informed decision about what puberty would be most appropriate for them. The Endocrine Society guidelines recommend clinicians inform and counsel all individuals seeking gender-affirming medical treatment regarding options for fertility preservation before initiating puberty suppression in adolescents and before treating with hormonal therapy of the affirmed gender in both adolescents and adults.[25]

In youth with gender dysphoria who have already started puberty, are beyond Tanner stage II, and have reached 16 years of age, the suggested medical treatment includes the use of hormone replacement therapy or gender-affirming hormones.[21,25] Gender-affirming hormones effectively cause the transgender youth to go through a second puberty, which brings about either the masculinization or feminization of their bodies and features. Because the sex hormones, estrogen and testosterone, are found in both natal males and natal females, providing hormone replacement therapy acts to rebalance the dominant hormone in the patient to match the patient's gender identity.

Because the transgender youth who are seeking treatment are minors, it is recommended that informed consent be obtained by a legal guardian, as well as assent (for adolescents) from the patient. Guardians and patients should be provided the information, education and resources to help them make informed decisions about the treatment options available to alleviate gender dysphoria and improve long-term health and mental health outcomes.

Aging and Elderly Patients

Like cisgender individuals, transgender people are subject to the vagaries of aging, and the potential conditions related to it. In general, screening and treatment of age-related illnesses in this population should be no different than in cisgender patients, with the exception of the use of appropriate organ inventories to guide screening. However, it is important to note that, for some transgender patients, it is only in later ages and stages of life that they feel safe to approach health care providers and others about their symptoms of gender dysphoria. Health care providers should be sensitive to, and have comfort with, discussing sexual orientation and gender identity issues with all aging patients. For transgender people who are aging, it is particularly important that primary care providers be familiar with the diagnosis of gender dysphoria and available treatments, including hormone therapy, mental health care, and surgical procedures. It is also important to address the potential for isolation and violence in the home as potential threats to aging transgender people.[45] A high index of suspicion for substance abuse, particularly alcohol use and misuse, is important. The combination of isolation, substance abuse, and depression can be particularly lethal for both cisgender and transgender elderly people, but the addition of stigma and the potential for violence and physical and mental abuse is particularly high among transgender individuals compared with their cisgender counterparts.[46] Overall, a high degree of compassion and sensitivity, combined with knowledge on the provider's part of current available therapies and best practices in medical record-keeping will help to ensure affirming care of aging transgender patients.

SUMMARY

As a growing number of transgender individuals become empowered to seek primary care, it is imperative that providers are prepared to meet their health care needs. This requires providers to approach these patient encounters with cultural humility and sound medical knowledge based on current guidelines. As new research emerges in the field of trans health clinicians will need to stay abreast of current best practices. In the meantime, clinicians could enhance care by creating a transgender-friendly office environment, conducting an annual organ inventory, updating their EHR system to incorporate transgender-friendly data collection, and taking into consideration current guidelines for gender affirmation, transition, screening, and prevention in this population.

REFERENCES

1. Spicer SS. Healthcare needs of the transgender homeless population. J Gay Lesbian Ment Health 2010;14(4):320–39.
2. Corliss HL, Shankle MD, Moyer MB. Research, curricula, and resources related to lesbian, gay, bisexual, and transgender health in US schools of public health. Am J Public Health 2007;97(6):1023–7.
3. Healthy People 2020. Lesbian, gay, bisexual, and transgender health. Available at: https://www.healthypeople.gov/2020/topics-objectives/topic/lesbian-gay-bisexual-and-transgender-health. Accessed December 4, 2017.

4. Jaime M. Grant PD, Mottet LA, et al. National transgender discrimination survey; report on health and healthcare. 2010.

5. Mizock L, Lewis T. Trauma in transgender populations: risk, resilience, and clinical care. J Emot Abuse 2008;8(3):335–54.

6. U.S. Transgender survey highlights disparities in healthcare access for trans Americans. 2016. Available at: https://nwlc.org/blog/u-s-transgender-survey-highlights-disparities-in-healthcare-access-for-trans-americans/. Accessed December 4, 2017.

7. Poteat T, German D, Kerrigan D. Managing uncertainty: a grounded theory of stigma in transgender health care encounters. Soc Sci Med 2013; 84(Supplement C):22–9.

8. Obedin-Maliver J, Goldsmith ES, Stewart L, et al. Lesbian, gay, bisexual, and transgender–related content in undergraduate medical education. JAMA 2011; 306(9):971–7.

9. Brown GR, Jones KT. Mental health and medical health disparities in 5135 transgender veterans receiving healthcare in the Veterans Health Administration: a case-control study. LGBT Health 2016;3(2):122–31.

10. Logie C, Bridge TJ, Bridge PD. Evaluating the phobias, attitudes, and cultural competence of master of social work students toward the LGBT populations. J Homosex 2007;53(4):201–21.

11. Kauth MR, Shipherd JC. Transforming a system: improving patient-centered care for sexual and gender minority veterans. LGBT Health 2016;3(3):177–9.

12. The Fenway Institute. Caring for LGBT older adults. Available at: https://www. lgbthealtheducation.org/wp-content/uploads/Caring-for-LGBT-Older-Adults.pdf. Accessed December 27, 2017.

13. Eliason MJ, Schope R. Original research: does "don't ask don't tell" apply to health care? lesbian, gay, and bisexual people's disclosure to health care providers. J Gay Lesbian Med Assoc 2001;5(4):125–34.

14. Sex, gender and sexual orientation in EPIC – strategy handbook. Verona (WI): EPIC; 2017.

15. Recommendations for inclusive data collection of trans people in HIV prevention, care & services. UCSF Center of Excellence for Transgender Health, San Francisco (CA). Available at: http://transhealth.ucsf.edu/trans?page=lib-data-collection. Accessed December 27, 2017.

16. Collecting sexual orientation and gender identity data in electronic health records. National LGBT Health Education Center. The Fenway Institute, Boston, MA. Available at: https://www.lgbthealtheducation.org/wp-content/uploads/ Collecting-Sexual-Orientation-and-Gender-Identity-Data-in-EHRs-2016.pdf. Accessed December 27, 2017.

17. Collazo A, Austin A, Craig SL. Facilitating transition among transgender clients: components of effective clinical practice. Clin Soc Work J 2013;41(3):228–37.

18. Auer MK, Fuss J, Höhne N, et al. Transgender transitioning and change of self-reported sexual orientation. PLoS One 2014;9(10):e110016.

19. Coleman E, Bockting W, Botzer M, et al. The Standards of Care (SOC) for the health of transsexual, transgender, and gender nonconforming people. Int J Transgend 2011;13:165.

20. White Hughto JM, Reisner SL. A systematic review of the effects of hormone therapy on psychological functioning and quality of life in transgender individuals. Transgend Health 2016;1(1):21–31.

21. Deutsch MB. Guidelines for the primary and gender-affirming care of transgender and gender nonbinary people. 2nd edition. UCSF; 2016. Available

at: http://transhealth.ucsf.edu/pdf/Transgender-PGACG-6-17-16.pdf. Accessed November 12, 2017.

22. Transgender health information program. Binding. Vancouver Coastal Health. Available at: http://transhealth.vch.ca/social-transition-options/binding-packingtucking/binding. Accessed November 12, 2017.

23. Dutton L, Koenig K, Fennie K. Gynecologic care of the female-to-male transgender man. J Midwifery Womens Health 2008;53(4):331–7.

24. Mepham N, Bouman WP, Arcelus J, et al. People with gender dysphoria who self-prescribe cross-sex hormones: prevalence, sources, and side effects knowledge. J Sex Med 2014;11(12):2995–3001.

25. Hembree WC, Cohen-Kettenis PT, Gooren L, et al. Endocrine treatment of gender-dysphoric/gender-incongruent persons: an endocrine society clinical practice guideline. J Clin Endocrinol Metab 2017;102(11):3869–903.

26. Misawa A, Inoue S. Estrogen-related receptors in breast cancer and prostate cancer. Front Endocrinol (Lausanne) 2015;6:83.

27. Gooren LJ, Giltay EJ, Bunck MC. Long-term treatment of transsexuals with cross-sex hormones: extensive personal experience. J Clin Endocrinol Metab 2008; 93(1):19–25.

28. Meyer WJ 3rd, Webb A, Stuart CA, et al. Physical and hormonal evaluation of transsexual patients: a longitudinal study. Arch Sex Behav 1986;15(2):121–38.

29. Bhasin S, Cunningham GR, Hayes FJ, et al. Testosterone therapy in men with androgen deficiency syndromes: an Endocrine Society clinical practice guideline. J Clin Endocrinol Metab 2010;95(6):2536–59.

30. Vesper HW, Botelho JC, Wang Y. Challenges and improvements in testosterone and estradiol testing. Asian J Androl 2014;16(2):178–84.

31. van Kesteren PJ, Asscheman H, Megens JA, et al. Mortality and morbidity in transsexual subjects treated with cross-sex hormones. Clin Endocrinol (Oxf) 1997;47(3):337–42.

32. Toorians AWFT, Thomassen MCLGD, Zweegman S, et al. Venous thrombosis and changes of hemostatic variables during cross-sex hormone treatment in transsexual people. J Clin Endocrinol Metab 2003;88(12):5723–9.

33. Cunha FS, Domenice S, Camara VL, et al. Diagnosis of prolactinoma in two male-to-female transsexual subjects following high-dose cross-sex hormone therapy. Andrologia 2015;47(6):680–4.

34. American Psychological Association. Guidelines for psychological practice with transgender and gender nonconforming people. Am Psychol 2015;70(9):832–64.

35. Simons L, Schrager SM, Clark LF, et al. Parental support and mental health among transgender adolescents. J Adolesc Health 2013;53(6):791–3.

36. Olson KR, Durwood L, DeMeules M, et al. Mental health of transgender children who are supported in their identities. Pediatrics 2016;137(3).

37. Lopez X, Stewart S, Jacobson-Dickman E. Approach to children and adolescents with gender dysphoria. Pediatr Rev 2016;37(3):89–98.

38. Horvath KJ, Iantaffi A, Swinburne-Romine R, et al. A comparison of mental health, substance use, and sexual risk behaviors between rural and non-rural transgender persons. J Homosex 2014;61(8):1117–30.

39. Hoy-Ellis CP, Fredriksen-Goldsen KI. Depression among transgender older adults: general and minority stress. Am J Community Psychol 2017;59(3–4):295–305.

40. Khatchadourian K, Amed S, Metzger DL. Clinical management of youth with gender dysphoria in Vancouver. J Pediatr 2014;164(4):906–11.

41. Almeida J, Johnson RM, Corliss HL, et al. Emotional distress among LGBT youth: the influence of perceived discrimination based on sexual orientation. J Youth Adolesc 2009;38(7):1001–14.

42. Clements-Nolle K, Marx R, Katz M. Attempted suicide among transgender persons: the influence of gender-based discrimination and victimization. J Homosex 2006;51(3):53–69.

43. Peterson CM, Matthews A, Copps-Smith E, et al. Suicidality, self-harm, and body dissatisfaction in transgender adolescents and emerging adults with gender dysphoria. Suicide Life Threat Behav 2017;47(4):475–82.

44. Costa R, Dunsford M, Skagerberg E, et al. Psychological support, puberty suppression, and psychosocial functioning in adolescents with gender dysphoria. J Sex Med 2015;12(11):2206–14.

45. Makadon HJ, Mayer KH, Potter J, et al. The Fenway guide to lesbian, gay, bisexual and transgender health. American College of Physicians; 2008.

46. Williams ME, Freeman PA. Transgender health: implications for aging and caregiving. J Gay Lesbian Soc Serv 2007;18(3–4):93–108.

47. Garofalo R, Wolf RC, Wissow LS, et al. Sexual orientation and risk of suicide attempts among a representative sample of youth. Arch Pediatr Adolesc Med 1999;153(5):487–93.

48. Díaz RM, Ayala G, Bein E, et al. The impact of homophobia, poverty, and racism on the mental health of gay and bisexual Latino men: findings from 3 US cities. Am J Public Health 2001;91(6):927–32.

49. Lim FA, Brown DV, Justin Kim SM. Addressing health care disparities in the lesbian, gay, bisexual, and transgender population. Am J Nurs 2014;114(6): 24–34.

50. Hafeez H, Zeshan M, Tahir MA, et al. Health care disparities among lesbian, gay, bisexual, and transgender youth: a literature review. Cureus 2017;9(4):e1184.

51. Substance Abuse and Mental Health Services Administration. Top health issues for LGBT populations information & resource kit. HHS Publication No. (SMA) 12-4684. Rockville (MD): Substance Abuse and Mental Health Services Administration; 2012.

52. Herbst JH, Jacobs ED, Finlayson TJ, et al. Estimating HIV prevalence and risk behaviors of transgender persons in the United States: a systematic review. AIDS Behav 2008;12(1):1–17.

53. Melendez RM, Exner TA, Ehrhardt AA, et al. Health and health care among male-to-female transgender persons who are HIV positive. Am J Public Health 2006; 96(6):1034–7.

54. Coulter RWS, Bersamin M, Russell ST, et al. The effects of gender- and sexuality-based harassment on lesbian, gay, bisexual, and transgender substance use disparities. J Adolesc Health 2017;62(6):688–700.

55. Edmiston EK, Donald CA, Sattler AR, et al. Opportunities and gaps in primary care preventative health services for transgender patients: a systemic review. Transgend Health 2016;1(1):216–30.

56. Gooren LJ. Management of female-to-male transgender persons: medical and surgical management, life expectancy. Curr Opin Endocrinol Diabetes Obes 2014;21(3):233–8.

57. Quinn GP, Sanchez JA, Sutton SK, et al. Cancer and lesbian, gay, bisexual, transgender/transsexual, and queer/questioning (LGBTQ) populations. CA Cancer J Clin 2015;65(5):384–400.

58. Hage JJ, Dekker JJ, Karim RB, et al. Ovarian cancer in female-to-male transsexuals: report of two cases. Gynecol Oncol 2000;76(3):413–5.

59. Dizon DS, Tejada-Berges T, Koelliker S, et al. Ovarian cancer associated with testosterone supplementation in a female-to-male transsexual patient. Gynecol Obstet Invest 2006;62(4):226–8.

60. Rogers TL, Emanuel K, Bradford J. Sexual minorities seeking services. J Lesbian Stud 2003;7(1):127–46.

Plastic Surgery for Women

Michelle M. De Souza, MD[a], Andrea D. Jewell, MD[b],
Samuel N. Grief, MD, FCFP[c], Belinda A. Vail, MD, MS[d],*

KEYWORDS

- Plastic surgery • Cosmetic surgery • Women • Breast surgery

KEY POINTS

- Face and brow lifts, eyelid surgery, and rhinoplasty are common facial cosmetic procedures performed on women, most to prevent or reverse the signs of aging.
- Injections of botulinum toxin and fillers and multiple types of lasers and pulsed light are now often used before surgery to even color and to induce collagen production, producing a smoother-appearing skin.
- Techniques for breast reconstruction after breast cancer surgery and breast reduction for macromastia are compared with the purely cosmetic procedures of augmentation and mastopexy.
- Liposuction is the most common cosmetic procedure performed on women, and it may also be combined with abdominoplasty or other procedures to provide contouring of the body.
- Labiaplasty and vulvar reconstruction have more recently become popular to enhance the appearance of the female genitalia.

Plastic surgery includes both reconstructive and cosmetic surgery. Derived from the Greek "plastikos" meaning to mold or give form, "plastic" surgery involves reconstruction, repair, or restoration of a deformity from a congenital defect, disease, or injury as well as cosmetic surgery for aesthetic improvement. The field is quite broad, but this article concentrates on cosmetic and breast procedures. Procedures vary considerably by age and gender (**Box 1**). Repair of congenital problems, especially maxillofacial procedures, are done primarily in children. More body contouring procedures, including liposuction and breast augmentation, are done in young women. As people age, procedures are performed in an attempt to reverse or delay the normal aging process with the current trend toward earlier procedures to delay signs of aging. Women

Disclosure Statement: The authors have nothing to disclose.
[a] Department of Plastic Surgery, University of Kansas School of Medicine, 3901 Rainbow Boulevard, Kansas City, KS 66160, USA; [b] Department of Obstetrics and Gynecology, University of Kansas School of Medicine, 3901 Rainbow Boulevard, Kansas City, KS 66160, USA; [c] Department of Family Medicine, University of Illinois at Chicago, Chicago, IL, USA; [d] Department of Family Medicine, University of Kansas School of Medicine, 3901 Rainbow Boulevard, Kansas City, KS 66160, USA
* Corresponding author. 3901 Rainbow Boulevard, Mailstop 4010, Kansas City, KS 66160.
E-mail address: bvail@kumc.edu

Prim Care Clin Office Pract 45 (2018) 705–717
https://doi.org/10.1016/j.pop.2018.07.008
0095-4543/18/© 2018 Elsevier Inc. All rights reserved.

Box 1
Most commonly performed procedures in 2016

The most commonly performed aesthetic procedures for women in 2016:

- Liposuction (369,323 procedures)
- Breast augmentation (310,444 procedures)
- Tummy tuck (173,536 procedures)
- Mastopexy (breast lift) (161,412 procedures)
- Eyelid surgery (145,858 procedures)

The most commonly performed aesthetic procedures for men in 2016:

- Liposuction (45,012 procedures)
- Breast reduction (31,368 procedures)
- Eyelid surgery (28,025 procedures)
- Nose surgery (26,205 procedures)
- Facelift (13,702 procedures)

The most common surgical procedures per age group in 2016:

- 18 and under: ear surgery
- 19 to 34: breast augmentation
- 35 to 64: liposuction
- 65 and over: eyelid surgery

Data from American Society for Aesthetic Plastic Surgery. Cosmetic surgery national data bank statistics. Available at: https://www.surgery.org/sites/default/files/ASAPS-Stats2016.pdf. Accessed October 15, 2017.

---

have traditionally been the most frequent consumers of cosmetic procedures, whereas men are more likely to be seen following injuries, but this demographic is changing as more men undergo cosmetic procedures.[1]

FACELIFT

A facelift, or rhytidectomy, is generally undertaken to improve visible signs of aging in the face and neck, including the following:

a. Relaxation of the skin of the face causing sagging
b. Deepening of the fold lines between the nose and corner of the mouth
c. Fat that has fallen or has disappeared
d. Jowls or the drooping lower portion of the cheeks
e. Loose skin and excess fat of the neck that can appear as a double chin or "turkey neck"

The number of surgeries performed has been increasing over the last 20 years, but a recent downturn is likely due to the increased use of less invasive procedures designed to restore a more youthful appearance by tightening skin and replenishing underlying soft tissue deficiency (atrophy and/or malposition) with fillers or fat grafting.[2]

Facelift is usually an outpatient procedure done under a range of anesthetics, depending on the extent of the surgery and patient and physician preference, from local anesthetic, to intravenous sedation, and occasionally general anesthesia.

There are several different techniques and varying degrees of the surgery, but most involve an incision along the temporal hairline extending in front, below, and behind the ears to the occipital hairline. The skin is separated from the underlying tissue, and in most cases, some skin is removed. The deeper connective tissue, known as the superficial musculo-aponeurotic system, is manipulated, usually by undermining or imbrication, to reposition the soft tissues deep to the skin in a more aesthetically favorable position.

A neck lift, also known as a lower rhytidectomy, impacts the neck and jaw areas.[3] An incision is made around the ears, and tightening of the platysma muscle (platysmaplasty) is undertaken, along with removal of any excess skin tissue. A submental incision may also be made to gain access to the medial border of the platysma muscle, allowing for additional manipulation and suturing. Redistribution and/or removal of a small amount of subcutaneous fat may also occur to enhance overall appearance and outcome.[3] Complications include hematomas, infections, nerve injuries, and skin flap ischemia. The skin and face will then continue the normal aging process, so these procedures are not expected to last a lifetime. Recovery from a facelift can be from a few days to weeks.

BROW LIFT

A brow lift, also known as a forehead lift or forehead rejuvenation, is a cosmetic surgical procedure to elevate the eyebrow region in patients with significant brow ptosis. Glabellar frown lines and forehead wrinkling can also be addressed with this procedure. It can be done through an endoscopic approach or through a larger coronal incision (hidden within the hairline at the junction of the frontal and parietal scalp or just in front of the hairline). A supraciliary (above the eyebrows) or within an existing forehead crease incision is also occasionally used and referred to as a "direct brow lift." It is usually done under general anesthetic. The most common problem is recurrent ptosis.

BLEPHAROPLASTY

Eyelid surgery, blepharoplasty, typically involves removing a small strip of redundant or sagging eyelid skin and underlying muscle, along with a variable amount of periobital fat, in order to return the upper and/or lower eyelid to a more youthful appearance.[4]

Excess eyelid skin, or dermatochalasis, typically accompanies the aging process explaining the high prevalence of this procedure in those over the age of 65. Dermatochalasis is the most common reason for upper lid blepharoplasty. It should not be confused with eyelid ptosis, which is an abnormality of the levator mechanism of the upper eyelid and results in a drooping lid. Complications of upper lid blepharoplasty include bleeding, injury to the levator mechanism resulting in ptosis, lacrimal gland injuries, and eye injuries. Lower lid blepharoplasty surgery can be done through a skin or conjunctival incision and is usually done to remove periorbital fat. A small amount of skin and/or orbicularis muscle may also be removed. Lower lids are more challenging and have a greater complication rate than upper lid blepharoplasty. Complications include hematoma, injuries to the extraocular muscles, ectropion, and blindness (very rarely). Good candidates for eyelid surgery include healthy, nonsmoking individuals who have no serious eye or health diseases.[5,6] These procedures are usually outpatient with a variety of anesthetics from local to general.

RHINOPLASTY

Cosmetic surgery of the nose involves both surgery on the nasal tip, primarily through manipulation of the cartilage, and surgery on the nasal bones, primarily narrowing of the nose by controlled fracture and manipulation. Rhinoplasty can also involve surgery on the nasal septum. Incisions can be made inside or outside the nose. Open rhinoplasty involves an incision across the columella. In closed rhinoplasty, the incisions are inside the nose at the level of the internal nasal valve. The procedure is usually done as an outpatient under general anesthesia. Complications include poor wound healing or scarring, septal perforation, and saddle deformity caused by lack of support from the nasal septum. Other problems are related to cosmetic irregularities and warping of the cartilaginous components of the nose. Considering reoperation to correct these problems is generally avoided until all edema has subsided, which can take up to 12 months.

INJECTABLES

Since the onset of the twenty-first century, minimally invasive aesthetic procedures have been championed as mitigating and cosmetically improving age-related facial changes.[7]

Injectable procedures are effective and tolerable with minimal to moderate discomfort and have a low incidence of adverse effects along with relatively short recovery times and rapid return to normal activity.[7] Injectables include botulinum toxin and dermal fillers.

Botulinum toxin (eg, onabotulinumtoxinA, Botox) is a potent neurotoxin originating from the bacterial species *Clostridium botulinum*.[7] It exerts its effect at the neuromuscular junction by inhibiting the release of acetylcholine, inducing temporary paralysis. Small quantities are injected into specific facial muscles, inducing muscle relaxation, resulting in smoother skin and visibly less wrinkles, and its injection is the most common nonsurgical cosmetic procedure.[1]

Botox was approved by the US Food and Drug Administration (FDA) for cosmetic use in 2002 to treat the glabellar complex muscles (corrugator and procerus muscles) that form frown lines,[8,9] and now has FDA approval to treat forehead (frontalis muscle) and periocular rhytids (orbicularis oculi muscle).[10,11]

A similar product, abobotulinumtoxinA (Dysport) was approved by the FDA in 2009 for the treatment of glabellar frown lines as well.[7] IncobotulinumtoxinA (Xeomin) was FDA-approved in 2010, originally for blepharospasm and then in 2011 for glabellar frown lines.[12]

Dermal fillers are injectable products administered to restore soft tissue volume for a defined period of time. They are the treatment of choice for facial lines and contour defects in the lower two-thirds of the face.[7,13] Bovine collagen was the first available type of filler, but risk of allergic reactions was high. Human collagen was also used, but has since been displaced by hyaluronic acid (HA) fillers due to HA's much longer duration of effect.[6,14] Other types of fillers include calcium hydroxylapatite and poly-L-lactic acid. The choice of which filler to use is related to their viscosity. The higher the viscosity, the longer they last, but they are more difficult to inject and are less forgiving. Use of fillers increased 10% in 2016 with the largest increase (16%) in HA injections.

Injection of autologous fat (fat grafting or transfer) has also become more popular to help augment soft tissues of the face where volume has been lost. Grafting involves harvesting fat, often from the abdomen or flanks, in the form of traditional liposuction. The fat is then prepared and immediately injected into the intended tissues. Advantages over the manmade products include availability of ample fat, contour improvement at the donor site, and longer lasting results. There is current interest in the adipose derived stem cells and their effect on the skin.

Complications of all injectables include injection site problems, infection, firmness/contour irregularity, and unpredictability of the injectable product. The most dreaded complication of injectable to the face is blindness due to the occlusion of the central retinal artery by retrograde injection of a fat emboli. Fortunately, this is extremely rare with about 47 reported cases through 2015[15]; however, prognosis for restoration of vision is poor.

MINIMALLY INVASIVE PROCEDURES

There are several laser treatments and other "minimally invasive" procedures available for patients that help to smooth fine lines and wrinkles and improve skin discoloration and texture. Fractional laser creates thousands of microscopic vertical channels of tissue destruction to induce collagen deposition as part of the healing process. This collagen deposition helps fill in the underlying tissue, producing a more youthful appearance by improving skin tone and texture, fine lines, and appearance of scars.

There are new hybrid fractional lasers on the market that deliver ablative and nonablative wavelengths to target different depths of the skin at the same time. Technology combines dermal rejuvenation with epidermal renewal to target sun damage to skin.

YAG lasers can address benign vascular lesions, port wine stains, rosacea, and hemangiomas.

Intense pulse light and broadband light treat a wide range of concerns, such as broken capillaries, age spots, discoloration, small veins, and rosacea.

Microlaser peel is an intraepidermal peel that precisely ablates the outermost layers of the skin. This peel treats many conditions, such as fine wrinkles, scars, keratosis, and discoloration.

Chemical peels are a process used to improve skin health by applying a chemical solution that causes the top layers of skin to separate and shed. A new, smooth, and youthful layer is revealed. Several popular formulations use trichloracetic acid, phenol, or glycolic acid as the base chemical with additives to enhance and control the depth of the peel.

Microneedling is a treatment designed to stimulate the skin's natural ability to repair itself, by creating a series of hundreds of vertical microscopic channels into the dermis, thus stimulating the natural production of new collagen and elastin.

BREAST
Augmentation

Breast augmentation has been the top cosmetic surgical procedure since 2006.[16] The goal for breast augmentation is to increase the size and or change the shape of a woman's breast primarily through the insertion of a breast implant. A successful breast augmentation surgery can boost a woman's confidence both with and without clothing.

There are several types of implants available in the United States. All have a silicone outer shell and are filled with either saline or a silicone gel. A highly cohesive silicone gel implant (referred to as a "gummy bear" implant) is more crosslinked and therefore is used to create a shaped implant or implants with more projection. They are all considered safe and are FDA approved and designed not to leak once the capsule is ruptured. The implants vary in size, surface texture, and shape, each with its own unique characteristics, advantages, and disadvantages. In the United States and across the world, silicone implants predominate. In 2016, silicone implants were used in 84%, and saline implants in 16%, of breast augmentations in the United States.[16]

Breast implants can be inserted under the muscle, under the breast gland, or under the fascia of the pectoralis muscle (subfascial). The incision location can be inframammary, periareolar, axillary, transabdominal (when combined with abdominoplasty), or umbilical (can only be done with saline implants which are inflated after placement).[17] Breast augmentation can be done in combination with a breast lift (mastopexy).

Autologous fat grafting for breast augmentation is a newer technique that is still being studied. Because not all grafted fat survives, the results are less predictable. Fat grafting for breast reconstruction is much more common and discussed later in this chapter.

Specific risks of breast augmentation include the following:

- Bleeding and infection
- Capsular contracture (abnormal scar tissue formation around the breast implant, varies from mild, to distortional, to painful)
- Implant failure (silicone shell breakage or silicone gel fracture)
- Implant malposition
- Breast implant–associated anaplastic large cell lymphoma (BIA-ALCL)[18]

Breast augmentation surgery will last several years; however, breast implants are not meant to be lifelong devices. For silicone breast implants, the FDA recommends MRI screening at 3 years and every 2 years thereafter to screen for implant failure.[19]

BIA-ALCL is a rare and highly treatable type of lymphoma that can develop around breast implants. BIA-ALCL occurs most frequently in patients who have breast implants with textured surfaces. According to the most recent data available, the lifetime risk of association between breast implants and ALCL is 1 in 30,000 patients with textured implants in the United States.[18]

Most of the patients who have developed BIA-ALCL receive an excellent prognosis following surgical removal of the breast implants and the surrounding capsule. Patients who notice pain, lumps, swelling, fluid collections or unexpected changes in breast shape, including asymmetry, should contact their plastic surgeon. In most cases, BIA-ALCL presents on average 8 to 10 years after receiving textured implants.[18]

Many women will seek or need additional surgeries for their breast implants. Some reasons for reoperation include implant failure, capsular contracture, implant malposition, desire for change in implant size, or because of changes to the breast over time.

Breast augmentation surgery is outpatient and typically done in an operating room with some level of anesthesia. The recovery for breast augmentation surgery is typically a few days for regular, activity, but vigorous activities may require more time. Drains are not typically placed.

Breast augmentation aside from breast reconstruction for cancer is not covered by insurance. Prices range for different surgeons, for different types of implants, and by geographic area. Quoted prices may or may not include anesthesia and facility fees.

Tuberous Breast Deformity

Tuberous breast deformity is a constricted breast development, usually bilateral, and characterized by a range of features[20]:

a. A contracted skin envelope both horizontally and vertically
b. A constricted breast base
c. A reduction in the volume of the breast parenchyma
d. Abnormal elevation of inframammary fold
e. Pseudoherniation of the breast parenchyma into the areola
f. Areola hypertrophy

The cause of tuberous breast is unclear. The pathogenesis of this breast deformity is linked to an aberration in thorax superficial fascia that blocks the normal expansion of glandular tissue.[20] Correction of the deformity is not necessary, but is often requested by women for aesthetic reasons.

Surgical goals for tuberous breast deformity are directed toward restoring volume (implants and/or fat grafting), reducing areola hypertrophy (skin reduction), lowering the inframammary fold, and expanding the lower pole skin envelope (implants, or adjacent tissue transfer techniques).

Mastopexy

Mastopexy "lifts" the woman's breasts with the goal of restoring a youthful appearance, typically after postpartum changes, with aging, or with weight loss. Ptosis is classified according to the position of the nipple in relation to the inframammary fold.[21] Correction involves separating the skin from the breast parenchyma and nipple, tightening the skin envelope, and raising the nipple in relation to the inframammary fold.

A spectrum of incisions may be used to lift the breasts. They range from periareolar (part way around the areola), circumareolar (all the way around the areola), circumareolar with an inferior vertical extension, to a full Wise pattern incision (inverted T or anchor). Larger breasts and those requiring greater lift will require larger incisions. The surgery is typically outpatient. Smaller breast lifts may be done in the office setting under local anesthesia.

For a woman who wants a breast lift with added volume, a breast implant can be added to the surgery, or staged into two surgeries, depending on patient factors and surgeon's preference. Combining the two surgeries increases the risks for complications, but is often requested by the patient.[22]

The results for a breast lift will last several years; however, with time, breast ptosis can recur. Significant changes in body habitus can also affect long-term results.

Mastopexy is not covered by insurance. Prices range for different surgeons, for different types of breast lift surgeries, and by geographic area.

Reduction

The goal for breast reduction surgery is to reduce the size and weight of a woman's breasts. Macromastia can cause back pain, neck pain, shoulder pain, inframammary rashes and moisture, bra strap grooving in the shoulders, and headaches, among other symptoms.

In addition to these signs and symptoms, insurance coverage also depends on the amount of weight to be removed from each breast. The amount is typically based on the patient's body surface area and can vary by insurance company. In addition, the woman should have failed nonsurgical options first, including weight loss, exercise, physical therapy, wearing supportive bras, chiropractic, use of pain relieving medications, strict hygiene, and prescribed medical treatment of any rashes.

Surgery will reduce the size of the breast as well as raise the position of the nipple areola complex. The incisions range from a vertical incision, to a vertical incision with a horizontal extension at or near the inframammary fold, to a full Wise pattern incision (inverted T or anchor). Liposuction alone can be used to reduce the volume of the breast, but this procedure may not be covered by insurance and raising the position of the nipple areola complex is not reliable. The surgery is either outpatient or extended recovery and may involve the use of postsurgical drains.

For most patients, the results are lifelong. However, breast size can change with significant weight gain or weight loss, with pregnancy, or with lactation. For a young woman having a breast reduction, it is important for her to know that she may need another breast reduction after pregnancy, lactation, or weight gain. Women should be counseled regarding the risks of surgery, including numbness or loss of the nipple areola complex, fat necrosis, and the potential inability to lactate.[23]

RECONSTRUCTION
Cancer

One in 8 women in the United States is diagnosed with breast cancer.[24] Surgery for breast cancer extirpation is common. A plastic surgeon is involved with re-creating the breast after a lumpectomy, partial mastectomy, or total mastectomy. The goal for breast reconstruction is to restore a woman's shape and form while in clothing. Restoring her breasts to a natural appearance while disrobed is a secondary goal.

Because of the Women's Health and Cancer Rights Act of 1998, federal law requires that a woman receiving benefits in connection with a mastectomy must also be provided benefits for the reconstruction and the contralateral breast balancing procedure.[25]

Breast reconstruction that is started at the time of the mastectomy is termed "immediate" reconstruction. Reconstruction that is begun after the mastectomy has healed is called "delayed" reconstruction.

Plastic surgeons reconstruct a breast using implants or autologous tissue. Breast reconstruction is often accomplished in multiple surgical stages. The first stage for many is the placement of a tissue expander. A tissue expander allows the surgeon to restore the size and shape of the breast envelope. The expander is filled with saline during subsequent office visits until the goal size is achieved. A second surgery is needed to remove the expander and place either a breast implant or autologous tissue. For selected patients, a breast reconstruction can be completed in a single stage at the time of mastectomy.

The need for chemotherapy and radiation will affect the decision making and possibly the results for a woman's breast reconstruction. The patient and her plastic surgeon should discuss her surgical options. The advantage of implant-based reconstruction is a simpler recovery without the need for an additional donor site. The main disadvantage is that implants are not intended to last a lifetime and infer the need for surgery in the future.

For autologous reconstruction, the main advantage is that the tissue has longevity. However, the surgery has a longer recovery, with the need to heal the donor site as well. Common pedicled autologous options are the latissimus dorsi myocutaneous flap or transverse rectus abdominus myocutaneous (TRAM) flap. With the advent of microsurgery, free tissue transfer options are now common,[26] to include the free TRAM flap, the deep inferior epigastric artery perforator flap, the superior inferior epigastric artery perforator flap, the transverse upper gracilis flap, the profundus artery perforator flap, the superior gluteal artery perforator flap, and the inferior gluteal artery perforator flap among others.

Autologous fat grafting is used as an adjunct or as a primary mode of breast reconstruction. It is accomplished by aspirating fat using liposuction, processing the fat in the operating room so that is ready for injection, and then grafting the fat into fine threads to allow the patient's blood supply to support the transplanted adipose tissue.

Congenital

Poland syndrome is characterized by an absence of the sternal head of the pectoralis muscle. Variable additional features include hypoplasia of the breast or nipple, scarcity of subcutaneous tissue, lack of the pectoralis minor muscle, aplasia or deformity of the costal cartilages of ribs II to IV or III to V, alopecia of the axillary and mammary region, and unilateral brachysyndactyly. It affects boys more than girls at a rate of 2:1 to 3:1. The incidence of Poland syndrome is 1 in 7000 to 1 in 100,000 live births.[27]

The goal for reconstructing of breast with Poland syndrome is to restore a breast shape. One feature that is distinct with this type of reconstruction is that a young girl's body will change throughout the course of the reconstruction and beyond.

Breast reconstruction for congenital amastia or Poland syndrome is done using either implants or autologous tissue or a combination of the two. It proceeds in a manner similar to breast cancer reconstruction. Coverage for congenital breast reconstruction varies by insurance company.

ABDOMINOPLASTY

The goal for an abdominoplasty is to restore abdominal contour and shape by tightening the skin, correcting rectus abdominus diastasis, and removing adiposity. Reasons that patients seek abdominoplasty include postpartum changes, rectus muscle diastasis, or changes to the abdomen after weight gain or loss. Intra-abdominal adiposity is not addressed with this surgery.

Concurrent with today's fashion trends, the typical placement of the abdominoplasty incision is low across the abdomen to be hidden within patient's clothing, most often extending from hip to hip. Liposuction can be used in combination with abdominoplasty to help contour the abdomen. The so-called mini-abdominoplasty may have a shorter scar, and the area of undermining and tissue repositioning is limited to the infraumbilical region.[28]

Patients are usually placed in a flexed "beach chair" position while in surgery to facilitate the removal of more abdominal tissue. The patient will take several days to walk upright until the tissue relaxes.

Recovery varies from patient to patient and depending on the extent of surgery. It can be difficult in the first 2 to 4 weeks after surgery due to pain, drains, and the flexed posture. Owing to the timeframe of collagen generation, there is no heavy lifting for 4 to 6 weeks. A postoperative garment is typically worn for days to weeks after surgery.

The results from abdominoplasty will last several years. Results can change with subsequent pregnancy or weight gain. Significant weight loss after abdominoplasty will contribute to additional skin laxity. For many patients, the improvement in abdominal contour can be confidence boosting, and clothing fits better.

For some patients, after massive weight loss, there is laxity in the anterior abdomen as well as the lower back and flanks. These patients will benefit from a circumferential abdominal approach, whereby the incision wraps from the front to the back of the patient. For some patients, the skin laxity is significant in both the vertical and the horizontal planes. These patients will benefit from a fleur-de-lis pattern excision, which results in both a vertical midline and a low horizontal incision. It is common for abdominoplasty patients to have drains, especially for larger surgeries, although some surgeons advocate for not using them.

Insurance does not typically cover abdominoplasty. Conversely, a panniculectomy, which is the removal of the redundant lower abdominal tissue that hangs over the pubis, is occasionally covered by insurance. The criteria for insurance coverage is frequent infra-pannicular rashes that require prescribed topical or oral antibiotics, and the excess abdominal skin must hang low enough to obscure at least the pubis, if not more, in an apron fashion. This pannus can interfere with ambulation and cause back pain.

Although the incisions are largely the same, a panniculectomy is distinct from an abdominoplasty by the extent of surgery. An abdominoplasty will address the whole abdomen whereas the panniculectomy only addresses the redundant overhanging tissue. Abdominoplasty can be either outpatient or extended recovery depending on the extent of surgery and patient factors.

LIPOSUCTION

Suction-assisted lipectomy, also known as liposuction, aims at reducing the adipose tissue in the subcutaneous space. In general, this procedure involves instilling tumescent solution into the subcutaneous tissue followed by aspiration of the fat using a blunt-tipped cannula.

The ideal liposuction patient has localized adiposity that has not been reduced by diet and exercise. However, with the safety and efficacy of liposuction, many people will use liposuction to debulk adiposity in large body mass index patients.

Adjuncts include laser-assisted, ultrasound-assisted, and power-assisted liposuction.[29] These forms of liposuction are modifications of the surgical technique; however, the overall surgical approach remains largely the same.

Many liposuction cases are outpatient. Large-volume liposuction cases may be observed overnight in a medical setting. The definition of large volume varies, but can be considered for a total aspirate that surpasses 4 or 5 L in one surgical procedure.[29] Results are expected to last lifelong if the patient maintains his or her weight. The adipocytes that are aspirated are permanently removed, but remaining adipocytes can enlarge with weight gain. Most patients note that with subsequent weight gain the fat is distributed to areas outside of the surgically treated area.

LABIAPLASTY AND VULVAR RECONSTRUCTION

Labiaplasty is becoming an increasingly popular cosmetic procedure in the United States with more than 8000 procedures performed in 2016.[30] Labiaplasty is defined as reduction of the labia minora. Terms such as "vaginal rejuvenation" are not recommended because it is medically unclear what procedure is being performed. There has been significant debate between the Plastic Surgery and Gynecology communities regarding the medical necessity and safety of such procedures.[31,32] Although most of the literature shows the procedure to be low risk and tolerated well by patients, it should be noted that most of the data is retrospective or noncomparative data.

Women undergo the procedure for various reasons, the most common being aesthetic, followed by functional impairment, and sexual concerns.[33] A prospective study of 50 patients undergoing the procedure showed that most women had multiple complaints related to both physical and aesthetic symptoms. These complaints included tugging during intercourse, twisting of labia, labia visible in tight pants, dyspareunia, concern for exposure in swimwear, and feeling self-conscious and less attractive.[32] Another study found that women seeking labiaplasty procedures had greater exposure to female genitalia on the Internet or through advertisements and were more likely to internalize these as standards for their own genitalia. Surprisingly, sexually active women seeking the procedure had similar sexual confidence, relationship quality, and self-esteem as their counterparts not seeking the procedure. However, significantly fewer women seeking the procedure were sexually active.[33] Therefore, it is important to adequately understand a patient's request for labiaplasty and provide education regarding the range of normal appearance in female genitalia and to discuss nonsurgical interventions.[34]

The procedure itself involves a range of techniques, including deepithelialization, direct excision wedge resection, and W- or Z-plasty procedures. At this time, there is no standard approach to labiaplasty. The primary goals for each procedure should be maintaining neurovascular supply, preserving the introitus, matching skin tones, and using the least invasive procedure to achieve reduction.[35] Complications are rare, with less than 7% rate noted in a large retrospective review, and patient satisfaction consistently exceeds 90%.[36] The most common complications are wound dehiscence, hematoma, bleeding, and urinary retention. A prospective trial sought to evaluate external genitalia sensitivity following labiaplasty and found that in the immediate postoperative period there was a diminished response; however, long term there was no significant altered sensitivity in either the labia or clitoral hood. Also, patients reported increases in sexual activity as well as orgasm frequency and strength.[37]

Ultimately, increasing popularity and high patient satisfaction will likely continue to increase the patient demand for labiaplasty. It is important to perform a complete history and physical examination to evaluate for possible body dysmorphic disorder and other physical findings that could be causing sexual dysfunction.

The other patient population to consider is the patient with vulvar dysplasia and cancer who undergoes resection and vulvar reconstruction. There is a wide variation of reconstruction available to this patient population. Patients who undergo radical surgery for vulvar cancer are at significantly increased risk of postoperative morbidity with more than 50% of patients with wound complications and upwards of 70% of patients with lymphedema.[38] Studies have shown that women experience significant psychosexual dysfunction following treatment of vulvar cancer, regardless of the extent of surgery.[39] It is recommended that a multidisciplinary approach be used, including physical therapy, counseling, consideration of hormone replacement therapy, and routine medical follow up.

ACKNOWLEDGMENTS

Richard J. Bene', MD; Paul Leahy, MD; Regina Nouhan, MD; Keith Hodge, MD: Monarch Plastic Surgery, private practice, 4801 West 135th Street, Leawood, KS 66224.

REFERENCES

1. Available at: https://www.surgery.org/sites/default/files/ASAPS-Stats2016.pdf. Accessed October 15, 2017.
2. Available at: https://www.plasticsurgery.org/cosmetic-procedures/facelift. Accessed October 15, 2017.
3. Available at: https://www.plasticsurgery.org/cosmetic-procedures/neck-lift. Accessed October 15, 2017.
4. Available at: https://www.plasticsurgery.org/cosmetic-procedures/eyelid-surgery/animation. Accessed October 15, 2017.
5. Available at: https://www.plasticsurgery.org/cosmetic-procedures/eyelid-surgery/procedure. Accessed October 15, 2017.
6. Available at: https://www.webmd.com/beauty/cosmetic-procedures-eyelid-surgery#1. Accessed November 1, 2017.
7. Small R. UCSF. Am Fam Physician 2009;80(11):1231–7.
8. Carruthers J, Carruthers A. The use of botulinum toxin type A in the upper face. Facial Plast Surg Clin North Am 2006;14(3):253–60.
9. Maas CS. Botulinum neurotoxins and injectable fillers: minimally invasive management of the aging upper face. Facial Plast Surg Clin North Am 2006;14(3):241–5.
10. Carruthers A, Carruthers J, Cohen J. A prospective, double-blind, randomized, parallel-group, dose-ranging study of botulinum toxin type A in female subjects with horizontal forehead rhytides. Dermatol Surg 2003;29(5):461–7.

11. Lowe NJ, Lask G, Yamauchi P, et al. Bilateral, double-blind, randomized comparison of 3 doses of botulinum toxin type A and placebo in patients with crow's feet. J Am Acad Dermatol 2002;47(6):834–40.

12. Available at: https://www.drugs.com/history/xeomin.html.

13. Wise JB, Greco T. Injectable treatments for the aging face. Facial Plast Surg 2006;22(2):140–6.

14. Fagien S, Klein AW. A brief overview and history of temporary fillers: evolution, advantages, and limitations. Plast Reconstr Surg 2007;120(6 suppl):8S–16S.

15. Belezenay K, Humphrey K, Humphrey S, et al. Avoiding and treating blindness from fillers: a review of the world literature. Dermatol Surg 2015;41(10):1097–117.

16. 2016 Complete plastic surgery statistics report. Available at: https://www.plasticsurgery.org/documents/News/Statistics/2016/plastic-surgery-statistics-full-report-2016.pdf. Accessed November 7, 2017.

17. David A, Hidalgo MD, Jason A, et al. Breast augmentation. Plast Reconstr Surg 2014;(133).

18. Information on BIA-ALCL. Available at: http://www.plasticsurgery.org/patient-safety/information-on-bia-alcl. Accessed November 7, 2017.

19. 2017. Available at: https://www.fda.gov/MedicalDevices/ProductsandMedical Procedures/ImplantsandProsthetics/BreastImplants/ucm064106.htm - Breast feeding. Accessed November 7, 2017.

20. Zoccali G, Giuliani M. Tuberous breast: clinical evaluation and surgical treatment. Current Concepts in Plastic Surgery 2012;135–53.

21. Regnault P. Breast ptosis: definition and treatment. Clin Plast Surg 1976;3:193–203.

22. Calobrace MB, Herdt DR, Cothron KJ. Simultaneous augmentation/mastopexy: a retrospective 5-year review of 332 consecutive cases. Plast Reconstr Surg 2013;(131):145–56.

23. Elizabeth J, Hall-Findlay MD, Kenneth C, et al. Breast reduction. Plast Reconstr Surg 2015;(136).

24. Cancer Statistics. Surveillance, epidemiology, and end results program. 2017. Available at: https://seer.cancer.gov/statfacts/html/breast.html. Accessed November 13, 2017.

25. The center for consumer information & insurance oversight. Available at: https://www.cms.gov/CCIIO/Programs-and-Initiatives/Other-Insurance-Protections/whcra_factsheet.html. Accessed November 13, 2017.

26. Serletti JM, Fosnot J, Nelson JA, et al. Breast reconstruction after breast cancer. Plast Reconstr Surg 2011;(127).

27. Alexander A, Fokin M, Francis Robicsek M. Poland's syndrome revisited. Ann Thorac Surg 2002;(74):2218–25.

28. Aly A. Abdominoplasty and lower truncal circumferential body contouring. 6th edition. Philadelphia: Lippincott Williams & Wilkins; 2007.

29. DeSouza M, II GM. Body contouring via suction lipectomy. In: Dayicioglu D, Oeltjen JC, Fan KL, et al, editors. Plastic reconstructive and aesthetic surgery the essentials. Singapore: World Scientific Publishing Co. Pte. Ltd.; 2012.

30. Sharp G, Tiggemann M, Mattiske J. A retrospective study of the psychological outcomes of labiaplasty. Aesthet Surg J 2017;37(3):324–31.

31. Pauls R, Rogers R. Should gynecologists provide cosmetic labiaplasty procedures? AJOG 2014;211(3):218–20.

32. Sorice SC, Li AY, Canales FL, et al. Why women request labiaplasty. Plast Reconstr Surg Glob Open 2016;139(4):856–63.

33. Sharp G, Tiggemann M, Mattiske J. Factors that influence the decision to undergo labiaplasty: media, relationships, and psychological well-being. Aesthet Surg J 2016;36(4):469–78.
34. ACOG Committee Opinion No. 378: vaginal "rejuvenation" and cosmetic vaginal procedures. Obstet Gynecol 2007;110(3):737–8.
35. Motakef S, Rodriguez-Feliz J, Chung MT, et al. Vaginal labiaplasty. Plast Reconstr Surg 2015;135(3):774–88.
36. Oranges CM, Sisti A, Sisti G. Labia minora reduction techniques: a comprehensive literature review. Aesthet Surg J 2015;35(4):419–31.
37. Placik OJ, Arkins JP. A prospective evaluation of female external genitalia sensitivity to pressure following labia minora reduction and clitoral hood reduction. Plast Reconstr Surg 2015;136(4):442e–52e.
38. Morrow CP. Morrow's gynecologic cancer surgery. 2nd edition. Encinitas (CA): South Coast Medical Publishing; 2013.
39. Green MS, Naumann R, Elliot M, et al. Sexual dysfunction following vulvectomy. Gynecol Oncol 2000;77(1):73–7.

Integrative Health for Women

Jennifer K. Phillips, MD[a],*, Stephanie A. Cockrell, LMSW, MSW[a],
Alisha N. Parada, MD[b]

KEYWORDS

- Integrative health • Integrative medicine (IM) • Self-care • Wellness
- Women's health • Complementary and alternative medicine (CAM) • Gender

KEY POINTS

- Integrative Medicine is a model of health care that combines both conventional and unconventional therapies that serve the whole person and focus on prevention and whole health.
- Women are the highest utilizers of health care and Integrative Medicine for a variety of reasons.
- Integrative Medicine represents a more "female energy" in the field of medicine, which is needed even more today as health care moves toward value-based care and out of high-cost and high-harm care.
- Integrative Medicine can be incorporated into medical practice and into health workers' lives for wellness. Primary care clinicians can bring Integrative Medicine to the general population through a variety of methods.

THE CHANGING LANDSCAPE OF THE UNITED STATES HEALTH CARE SYSTEM

The American health care system has undergone drastic changes in the past 100 years and continues to evolve. The success of conventional medicine cannot be denied. However, these advances have led to an expensive and fragmented health care system, in which technology has eroded the patient-provider relationship. Patients are often shuffled between specialists, encouraged to believe drugs, tools, and technology are the answer to all problems. Medical care is directed at pieces of the patient's problem, rather than the whole person. It is not surprising that research strongly demonstrates that Americans are dissatisfied with their health care experiences. Patients are demanding choices in their health care, have a growing interest in nontraditional health care services, and have awareness of the interplay between the body, mind, community, and spirit.

Disclosure: The authors have nothing to disclose.
[a] Department of Family and Community Medicine, University of New Mexico, 2400 Tucker Boulevard Northeast, MSC09 5040, Albuquerque, NM 87131-0001, USA; [b] Department of Internal Medicine, University of New Mexico School of Medicine, UNM Health Sciences Center, 1 University of New Mexico, MSC10 5550, Albuquerque, NM 87131-0001, USA
* Corresponding author.
E-mail address: jkphillips@salud.unm.edu

Prim Care Clin Office Pract 45 (2018) 719–729
https://doi.org/10.1016/j.pop.2018.07.009
0095-4543/18/Published by Elsevier Inc.

primarycare.theclinics.com

WOMEN AND HEALTH

The health of women in the United States is subject to wide disparities. Women suffer from certain health conditions more than men, including breast cancer and stroke, but they are also more likely to die after a heart attack and are less likely to be treated for high cholesterol. Women are more likely to report having stress and say that their stress has increased over the last 5 years.[1] Women are less likely to be able to get medical care, dental care, and needed prescription medications.[2]

Women are the biggest consumers of health care. They have traditionally been the caregivers for their families and often drive the medical choices. Women may prefer health care that is higher "touch" and lower "tech." They have been shown to highly value connection with their health care providers and desire more autonomy and choice in their health care decisions. These factors, among others, have led to a surge of interest in complementary and alternative medicine (CAM) among the general population and especially in women.

USE OF INTEGRATIVE MEDICINE/COMPLEMENTARY AND ALTERNATIVE MEDICINE

The fragmented health care system, patient's dissatisfaction with their health care experiences, and a growing awareness of whole person health has contributed to the significant interest in and growing utilization of CAM. Multiple large-scale surveys of CAM use in the United States have been conducted, including data from the 2002, 2007, and 2012 Adult Alternative Medicine supplement to the National Health Interview Surveys.[3] Among US adults, "the prevalence of CAM use in the past 12 months" ranged from 32.3% in 2002 to 35.5% in 2007 and was most recently 33.2% in 2012. These results are consistent with previous research.[3] Although the percentage of usage declined slightly in 2012, it is important to note that this may be due to the lack of standardized guidelines regarding which CAM approaches are included in the surveys, and these definitions have narrowed over time.

EVOLUTION OF TERMINOLOGY/DEFINITIONS

Numerous terms have been used when referring to medical therapies outside of conventional medicine, due largely to the difficulty in developing a single, agreed upon term and definition. A 2016 textual analysis of the shifts in terminology between 1975 and 2013 revealed the most commonly used terms as "complimentary," "alternative," and "integrative."[4] The Complementary can be confusing and interrelated. Many of these terms are used to describe unconventional medicine in North America. As defined by the National Center for Complementary and Integrative Health, "complementary" is defined as a nonmainstream practice used together with conventional medicine and "alternative" as a nonmainstream practice used in place of conventional medicine. Complementary and Alternative Medicine (CAM) is a term used to describe modalities and treatments of nonmainstream origin. Although related, the use and definition of "integrative" medicine are unique, including a new model of health care that combines both conventional and unconventional therapies that serve the whole person and focus on prevention and maintenance of health, using evidence to understand how best to combine these therapies (**Fig. 1**).[4]

Integrative medicine has also been described as: "Healing oriented and emphasizes the centrality of the doctor patient relationship. It focuses on the least

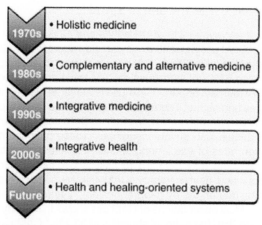

Fig. 1. Evolution of titles in the field. (*From* Rakel D, Weil A. Philosophy of integrative medicine. In: Rakel D, editor. Integrative medicine, 4th edition. Philadelphia: Elsevier Health Sciences; 2017. p. 2–12; with permission.)

invasive, least toxic and least costly methods to help facilitate health by integrating both allopathic and complementary therapies. These are recommended based on an understanding of the physical, emotional, psychological and spiritual aspects of the individual."[5] Integrative medicine emphasizes the use of evidence to understand how best to integrate CAM therapies into health care. There has also been an evolution away from the term integrative medicine to integrative health, which emphasizes the importance of the process of achieving whole health and health outcomes (**Fig. 2**).

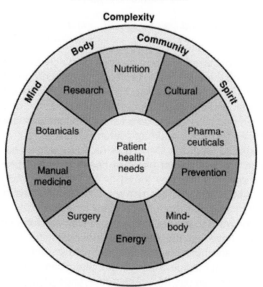

Fig. 2. Integrative medicine pie chart. (*From* Rakel D, Weil A. Philosophy of integrative medicine. In: Rakel D, editor. Integrative medicine, 4th edition. Philadelphia: Elsevier Health Sciences; 2017. p. 2–12; with permission.)

INTEGRATIVE MEDICINE USE IN THE UNITED STATES

According to a 2012 survey, 33.2% of US adults and 12% of US children are using some form of CAM.[3] CAM use by all 40 to 50 year olds nears 50%.[6] CAM use in Native American and Alaska Natives is 50.3%. CAM use is estimated to be significantly higher in rural areas, reaching 63%.[7] National use of CAM is estimated to be highest in New Mexico and the US Mountain region.[7] CAM use is higher in elderly as well as people with a college degree and higher. There are multiple studies that support the idea that wealthy populations use CAM the most. In studies, CAM use has also been shown to be highest among people with private insurance.[6] These data seem to conflict with studies showing high rates of use among Native American populations and people in rural areas. These data may be hard to assess because of language barriers, geographic variation, and health literacy. CAM use by socioeconomic status and ethnicity seems to be moderated by geographic region, and this needs to be studied further. For instance, local observations of CAM use shows that it may be higher in Hispanics in New Mexico than the national statistics of 23.7%.[7] CAM use is very likely to be influenced by cultural heritage and ethnic subgroups.

Demographics are not the only factor. Specific attitudes and beliefs seem to influence CAM use in patients with cancer.[8] Most evidence around CAM use is from oncology literature, and evidence is lacking in other areas. There are limited data about what really influences CAM use, and more studies need to be done to better understand these trends. Some survey research found that postmodern values like beliefs in natural healing, rejection of authority, and a desire for control can predict positive attitudes about CAM.[9,10]

WOMEN'S USE OF INTEGRATIVE MEDICINE AND INFLUENCE ON MEDICINE IN GENERAL

Women have always been healers. Medicine is part of our heritage as women, our history, our birthright.
– Barbara Ehrenreich and Deirdre English, Witches, Midwives, and Nurses:
A History of Women Healers[11]

Many changes have occurred in modern health care now that more women are in the field of medicine and the allied health professions. Not only are there more women doctors and clinicians of all types but also they have leadership and prescriptive authority, which has changed the direction of many areas of medicine. One must also consider the changes that have been made to modern medicine because of feminine consumer demand; that is, in the realm of "natural childbirth."[12]

The realm of Integrated Medicine (IM) is dominated by women as either patients or providers.[13] Women are the highest users of health care and preventive care and CAM. Women represent the majority (60%) of all CAM use, and they are 3 times more likely to use CAM than men.[14] Women are also the most health-aware members of society. They often seek out more health care for themselves than men and are more likely to look for ways to maintain health and wellness for themselves and their families.[14,15] Women have led the consumer movement for Integrative Medicine perhaps because they are more open to natural therapies, mind-body interventions, and healing traditions from outside "mainstream" American culture.[16]

As many as 75% of women use IM.[17] There is a range of 50% to 82% of reported CAM use in women for specific conditions.[14,17,18] Compared with male CAM users, women CAM users are more likely to have a bachelor's degree, be divorced, be separated or widowed, and be less likely to earn $75,000 a year or more. When comparing men and women CAM users, there are no differences between age, region, race, ethnicity, and family medical expense.[14] Women CAM users are more likely to use one or more modalities. Back pain is the top health condition that both men and women use CAM. "Other nonspecified conditions" is the second most reported health condition for which CAM is used.[14]

There are many gender-specific health experiences that women use CAM for, including pregnancy, premenstrual syndrome, menstruation, perimenopause, and postmenopause. There are also gender-specific health issues, including chronic pelvic pain, vulvodynia, vaginitis, and endometriosis for which CAM is used.[17]

TOP TYPE OF COMPLEMENTARY AND ALTERNATIVE MEDICINE THERAPIES USED BY ALL UNITED STATES ADULTS

Of the top 10 health conditions, there are only 2 that vary between men and women (**Fig. 3**). Chronic pain and stomach issues were higher for male CAM users, and headache or migraine and frequent stress were higher in female CAM users.[14]

UNPACKING THE FACTORS ASSOCIATED WITH COMPLEMENTARY AND ALTERNATIVE MEDICINE USE BETWEEN MEN AND WOMEN

Motivations to use CAM differ between men and women. Women are more likely to report positive outcomes from CAM use. Women state they are motivated to use CAM to improve general wellness, for general disease prevention, and to improve their overall health and well-being.[14] Women more often use CAM to maintain health or create "wellness." Wellness is defined as having a positive emotional state, regardless of health status or disease burden.[12] Maintenance of wellness involves healthy diet, regular exercise, getting enough and good quality sleep, stress reduction, massage, mindfulness, and spirituality to name just some of the factors.

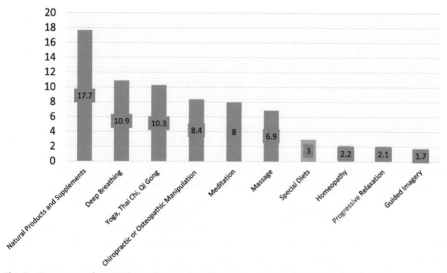

Fig. 3. Top types of CAM therapies used by US adults. (*Data from* Barnes PM, Bloom B, Nahin R. CDC national health statistics report #12. In: Complementary and alternative medicine use among adults and children: United States, 2007. December 2008. Available at: nccih.nih.gov/news/camstats/. Accessed October 20, 2017.)

Men often use CAM to improve athletic or sports performance. Men have been noted to use CAM in pursuit of lost masculinity or to improve virility, so using CAM may be perceived as a sign of weakness or impotence.[14] Men may interpret the need for wellness as problematic; it may seem like a need to maintain wellness weakens their masculinity. Women view maintaining wellness more positively. When women seek wellness by using CAM, it may be more socially acceptable. More holistic care also aligns with women's needs for autonomy in health care decisions and a need to be heard by their health care provider.[14] Women may seek empowerment and a connection with their provider and may find this more often with CAM.

Some research has suggested that women's use of CAM must not be perceived as female empowerment, and men's use of CAM cannot be seen as a challenge to conventional masculinity because in their study men and women enjoyed CAM through their own "gender lenses."[19] In this study, men often used CAM emphasizing science and rationality, while rejecting aspects of CAM that they saw as more feminine or emotional. Men often would discuss their CAM use in terms of postmodern or neoliberal values like self-reinvention, self-control, and being an informed consumer. Women would often discuss their CAM use to address problems with abusive relationships, low self-esteem, and body image concerns.[19]

THEORIES OF PHYSIOLOGY, BELIEF MANAGEMENT, AND DESIRE FOR CONTROL IN COMPLEMENTARY AND ALTERNATIVE MEDICINE USE

Physiology has been used to explain why women use CAM more. It is thought that men may respond to stress and illness with a "fight-or-flight" response, and it has been theorized that women release more oxytocin in times of stress and more often "tend and befriend." This oxytocin release may cause women to search out a practitioner when sick with whom they feel more connected.. Emotional connections are especially important to women, and women may seek more meaningful interactions with their health care providers. Western medicine may be too disease focused and often can dismiss the psychosocial aspects of illness and health.

Theories are increasingly being used to understand the complex, numerous factors associated with increased prevalence of CAM use. The Theory of Planned Behavior (TPB) implies that an individual chooses a particular behavior based on 3 major components: the patient's attitude toward the behavior (eg, perceived effectiveness of CAM therapies), perceived control (eg, individual's perception related to the difficulty of engaging in the new behavior), and subjective norms (eg, expectations from family and cultural views regarding CAM).[20] There is considerable support for TPB, which has been used as a theoretic framework to predict intention and behavior in a wide range of health-related behaviors. In 2015, Bauml and colleagues[8] applied TPB to CAM utilization and found that TPB was predictive of CAM use; more specifically they found that attitudes and beliefs accounted for more variance in CAM use than clinical and demographic factors alone. This finding may further explain women's increased CAM utilization because research demonstrates that women have more positive beliefs about CAM therapies and their effectiveness.[14]

Among patients with cancer, women use CAM more than men. Researchers have theorized that this is due to differences in how women cope with a cancer diagnosis.[18] People with cancer often feel a loss of control, and both women and men may seek alternative therapies that help them regain this sense of control. In one study 65% of women and 35% of men had a high desire for control.[18] Some research has found that men with serious and potentially fatal conditions like cancer are more accepting of the emotional and physical benefits of CAM use.[21]

"MASCULINE" AND "FEMININE" ENERGIES

Some investigators have gone so far as to describe Integrative Medicine as a "socially feminized" form of health care that does not have the same scientific legitimacy as standard biomedical practice.[13] Some have suggested that women's participation in Integrative Medicine, as practitioners and users, may reinforce women's second class or subordinate status and that of Integrative Medicine.[22]

It is true that medicine in the past has been dominated by more "masculine energy," and with the increasing interest in Integrative Medicine, there has been a swing toward more balance between the "female" and "male" energies. In the past, "feminine" qualities have been undervalued and oppressed in societies all over the world.

However, the world is changing, and those who embrace both "masculine" and "feminine" energies in balance will be the most successful. In an interview with John Gerzema, the author of the *Athena Doctrine*, he says, "The most effective leaders right now—men and women—are those who embrace traits once considered feminine: Empathy. Vulnerability. Humility. Inclusiveness. Generosity. Balance. Patience." He goes on to say, "Feminine traits and values are a new form of innovation." This need for more feminine energy has become apparent in health care as well, with a drive for more quality and value in health care experiences. in health care experiences. Health and healing have been long associated with the "female energy," and disciplines like medicine and surgery where there is a "find it fix it" mentality have been associated with "male energy."[23] Efforts to improve and focus on quality and patient satisfaction may be seen as "soft science" but are known to improve patient experience, increase compliance and decrease litigation.

STATISTICS OF DISCLOSURE AND NONDISCLOSURE OF COMPLEMENTARY AND ALTERNATIVE MEDICINE USE

There are numerous studies documenting a lack of communication between patients and their primary care clinicians about patients' use of CAM. National studies have found about 60% of those using CAM report never discussing it with their clinician. There may be more nondisclosure by certain ethnicities, with the highest rate of nondisclosure in Hispanics at 68%, followed by non-Hispanic blacks at 65%, and non-Hispanic whites at 58% in one study.[24]

One study found that more than half of clinicians have negative attitudes about CAM when they talked to their patients about it, and most felt uncomfortable during the discussions. Not surprisingly, the more physicians knew about CAM options, the more comfortable they felt discussing it with their patients.[25] Patient data suggest clinician initiation, when carried out in a nonjudgmental fashion, would help patients overcome anticipated or previous negative interactions in discussions about CAM, and patients usually did not expect their clinicians to be CAM experts.[25]

These data underscore the importance of the clinician's role in conversation initiation and comprehensive assessment of CAM utilization and whole person-centered health. Patients expect and welcome these discussions. Clinicians do not need to be CAM experts; rather a nonjudgmental interest and collaborative conversation are most important. It is particularly important for CAM use to be a routine part of a medication history because many of the herbs, supplements, and other CAM treatments people turn to could have potentially dangerous interactions with conventional therapies, particularly pharmaceutical medications.[25] Researchers suggest brief communication trainings for clinicians could have a significant impact in improving these conversations.[26]

When assessing, one can start by asking these basic questions: "What vitamins, minerals, and supplements are you taking? What prior experience have you had with integrative, complementary, or alternative medicine? What do you do to relax? What are the major stressors in your life and how do you deal with them?"

HOW TO BRING INTEGRATIVE MEDICINE INTO YOUR PRACTICE AND LIFE

As the demand for Integrative Medicine and expanded therapeutic approaches increases, health care providers find themselves asking "what can I do to learn more?"

Education is now being offered at all stages of medical education. There are now courses and curriculum that are offered but not limited to medical school and postgraduate training. There are computer-based curricula available online and fellowship programs that cater to health workers of all types. Board certification is available to physicians after completing a qualifying fellowship program, and there are several certificate programs for other allied health professionals. The Arizona Center for Integrative Medicine has training programs for health care professionals emphasizing health coaching and core concepts in IM.[27] To review the certification requirements to become certified by the American Board of Integrative Medicine, please visit the link below. This link also has information about the American Board of Integrative Medicine–approved fellowships, which are available across the country. The link to Integrative Medicine Fellowships is http://www.abpsus.org/integrative-medicine-fellowships.[28]

HEALTH WORKER WELLNESS

It is important to remember that in order to take care of others, health care workers need to care for themselves. Self-care as a medical provider is often overlooked and "trained away" during conventional medical training. If you are reading this article, you are likely looking for guidance on how to not only help improve the care of your patients, but also to improve your own health and well-being.

Health care workers of all types can start by taking wellness inventories like the Maslach burn-out inventory[29] or the "Mini-z"[30] in order to better assess their own wellness and self-care. We are currently practicing in a high burnout profession, and clinicians are leaving medicine at alarming rates. Unfortunately, burnout and suicide in clinicians are too common, and thankfully, there is now more attention being brought to this topic.

Integrative Medicine training provides important, essential skills that are not traditionally taught during medical training. Concepts and skills such as motivational interviewing can completely change how a health worker approaches patients and outcomes. Learning communication and motivational interviewing skills can also improve a health workers' satisfaction with their work. Integrative Medicine training also teaches reflective and self-care practices to the health care worker, which commonly changes their approach to providing care to others.

Asking questions like "what brings you joy?" or "what do you like about being alive?" or "what makes life worth living?" is a way to get at the whole story of a person's life. Exploring a person's particular beliefs can change the dynamic between patient and provider. Being more patient-centered and incorporating patient goals into health care conversations and the electronic health record can be meaningful to both patients and their providers. Integrative Medicine can help get to the cause of the cause and the "root" of illness. For those in primary care, it is an incremental journey with patients and their health and wellness.[31] It is important and powerful to help patients understand that one must avoid disease by avoiding its causes, and it is best to try the simple remedies before using the complex. Integrative medicine's simplicity can save lives, trouble and money.

Clinicians who integrate complementary therapies into their practice have decreased referrals and lower treatment costs.[32] Integrating these practices into your life and work can help improve personal resilience of health workers' and patients and help create a culture of wellness that, along with efficiency of practice, can be drivers of health worker wellness. Healthy clinicians give better care. They are known to have decreased medical errors, have increased patient satisfaction, give better and more thorough treatment recommendations, and have increased treatment adherence, lower malpractice risk, better attitudes toward work, higher team functioning, and lower turnover.[33]

Health worker wellness is important and needs a multipronged approach. Health system wellness is beyond the scope of this article but is related to health worker wellness. Burnout rates in medicine are at an all-time high, and ease and joy of practice with systemic changes in the health care system are needed along with individual resilience and wellness. Health care workers working in multidisciplinary teams to care for patients can also take off some of the burden that is associated with being a solo physician in practice. Health care workers can be powerful examples for patients, and trying these simple methods and helping others with them as well can be transformative.

SUMMARY

As the "female" and "male" energy becomes more balanced on the planet, the need for more holistic and value-based health care is becoming more apparent. Integrative Medicine and Health is more popular, and the demand for it is increasing in the general population and especially among women. It can be integrated into primary care and other health care fields and used by health care workers to improve the health and well-being of patients and themselves.

There are critics who argue that Integrative Medicine "provides individualistic solutions to problems of health by focusing on changing the individual rather than on altering the social structure that promotes an unhealthful environment."[34] This oversimplification of Integrative Medicine creates a false dichotomy, as individual approaches as well as societal approaches are important to improve health. Health care policy must focus on the systems that create disease and the social determinants of health. Individual care must focus on addressing individual social determinants of health, prevention, and treatments that are simple, and modalities and tools that increase wellness and health.

Optimum health and wellness are 2 different things. Health care workers must strive for the health of the population by improving the health system and increasing justice and reducing disparities. Individuals must strive for wellness, which is to have a positive emotional state, regardless of health status or disease burden. The goal is to live the fullest and most wonderful lives, meeting the deepest needs of being one with humanity and the planet and in service to both.

REFERENCES

1. National Institutes of Health. What health issues or conditions affect women differently than men? In NIH Health & Research Topics. Available at: https://www.nichd.nih.gov/health/topics/womenshealth/conditioninfo/pages/howconditions.aspx. Accessed November 27, 2017.
2. Agency for Healthcare Research and Quality. Healthcare quality and disparities in women: selected findings from the 2010 National Healthcare Quality and Disparities Reports. 2014. Available at: http://archive.ahrq.gov/research/findings/nhqrdr/nhqrdr10/women.html. Accessed November 17, 2017.
3. Clarke TC, Black LI, Stussman BJ, et al. Trends in the use of complementary health approaches among adults: United States, 2002-2012. Natl Health Stat Report 2015;(79):1–16.

4. Ng JY, Boon HS, Thompson AK, et al. Making sense of "alternative", "complementary", "unconventional" and "integrative" medicine: exploring the terms and meanings through a textual analysis. BMC Complement Altern Med 2016;16:134.

5. Rakel D, Weil A. Philosophy of integrative medicine. In: Rakel D, Their SO, editors. Integrative medicine. 4th edition. Philadelphia (PA): Elsevier Health Sciences; 2017. p. 2–12.

6. Barnes PM, Bloom B, Nahin R. CDC National Health Statistics Report #12. In: complementary and alternative medicine use among adults and children: United States, 2007. 2008. Available at: nccih.nih.gov/news/camstats/. Accessed October 20, 2017.

7. Marshik PL, Kharat AA, Jakeman B, et al. Complementary and alternative medicine and therapy use in a diverse New Mexican population. J Altern Complement Med 2015;22(1):45–51.

8. Bauml JM, Chokshi S, Schapira MM, et al. Do attitudes and beliefs regarding complementary and alternative medicine impact its use among patients with cancer? A cross-sectional survey. Cancer 2015;121(14):2431–8.

9. Rayner L, Easthope G. Postmodern consumption and alternative medications. J Sociol 2001;37(2):157–76.

10. Siahpush M. Postmodern values, dissatisfaction with conventional medicine and popularity of alternative therapies. J Sociol 1998;34(1):58–70.

11. Low Dog T, Maizes V. Women's health: epilogue. In: Maizes V, Low Dog T, Their SO, editors. Integrative women's health. 2nd edition. New York: Oxford University Press; 2015. p. 808–15.

12. Hudson T. Women's encyclopedia of natural medicine: alternative therapies and integrative medicine for total health and wellness. 2nd edition. New York: McGraw-Hill Education; 2007. xviii–xvii.

13. Sointu E. Detraditionalisation, gender and alternative and complementary medicines. Sociol Health Illn 2011;33(3):356–71.

14. Zhang Y, Leach MJ, Hall H, et al. Differences between male and female consumers of complementary and alternative medicine in a National US population: a secondary analysis of 2012 NIHS data. Evid Based Complement Alternat Med 2015;2015:413173.

15. Vaidya V, Partha G, Karmakar M. Gender differences in utilization of preventive care services in the United States. J Womens Health (Larchmt) 2012;21(2):140–5.

16. Weil A. Forward. In: Maizes V, Low Dog T, Their SO, editors. Integrative women's health. 2nd edition. New York: Oxford University Press; 2015. ix–xii.

17. Chiaramonte D, Ring M, Locke AB. Integrative women's health. Med Clin North Am 2017;101(5):955–75.

18. Hedderson MM, Patterson RE, Neuhouser ML, et al. Sex differences in motives for use of complementary and alternative medicine among cancer patients. Altern Ther Health Med 2004;10(5):58–64.

19. Brenton J, Elliott S. Undoing gender? The case of complementary and alternative medicine. Sociol Health Illn 2014;36(1):91–107.

20. Hirai K, Komura K, Tokoro A, et al. Psychological and behavioral mechanisms influencing the use of complementary and alternative medicine (CAM) in cancer patients. Ann Oncol 2008;19(1):49–55.

21. Evans M, Shaw A, Thompson EA, et al. Decisions to use complementary and alternative medicine (CAM) by male cancer patients: information-seeking roles and types of evidence used. BMC Complement Altern Med 2007;7:25.

22. Flesch H. Silent voices: women, complementary medicine, and the co-optation of change. Complement Ther Clin Pract 2007;13(3):166–73.

23. Buchanan L. Between venus and mars: 7 traits of true leaders. Available at: https://www.inc.com/magazine/201306/leigh-buchanan/traits-of-true-leaders.html. Accessed November 27, 2017.
24. Graham RE, Ahn AC, Davis RB, et al. Use of complementary and alternative medical therapies among racial and ethnic minority adults: results from the 2002 National Health Interview Survey. J Natl Med Assoc 2005;97(4):535–45.
25. National Women's Health Report: complementary & alternative medicine for women in: healthy women. Available at: http://www.healthywomen.org/content/publication/national-womens-health-report-complementary-alternative-medicine-women. Accessed November 29, 2017.
26. Shelley BM, Sussman AL, Williams RL, et al, Clinicians on behalf of the RN. 'They Don't Ask Me So I Don't Tell Them': patient-clinician communication about traditional, complementary, and alternative medicine. Ann Fam Med 2009;7(2):139–47.
27. The University of Arizona Center for Integrative Medicine. Education courses and Programs. Available at: https://www.integrativemedicine.arizona.edu/education/index.html. Accessed October 20, 2017.
28. Integrative medicine fellowships. Available at: http://www.abpsus.org/integrative-medicine-fellowships. Accessed November 29, 2017.
29. Maslach C, Jackson SE, Leiter MP. Maslach burnout inventory manual. 3rd edition. Palo Alto (CA): Consulting Psychologists Press; 1996 (577 College Ave., Palo Alto 94306).
30. Linzer M. Mini Z burnout survey. Available at: https://www.stepsforward.org/modules/physician-burnout-survey. Accessed November 27, 2017.
31. Gawande A. The heroism of incremental care. In: The New Yorker. 2017. Available at: https://www.newyorker.com/magazine/2017/01/23/the-heroism-of-incremental-care. Accessed November 2, 2017.
32. White AR, Ernst E. Economic analysis of complementary medicine: a systematic review. Complement Ther Med 2000;8(2):111–8.
33. Federation of state medical boards. Available at: http://www.fsmb.org. Accessed November 27, 2017.
34. McKee J. Holistic health and the critique of Western medicine. Soc Sci Med 1988; 26(8):775–84.

Medication-Assisted Treatment Considerations for Women with Opiate Addiction Disorders

Alicia A. Jacobs, MD*, Michelle Cangiano, MD

KEYWORDS

- Opioid-use disorder (OUD) • Opioid addiction • Medication-assisted therapy (MAT)
- Trauma-informed care • Buprenorphine • Hub-and-spoke model • Harm reduction

KEY POINTS

- Rates of opioid-use disorder (OUD) and its adverse outcomes are skyrocketing in women.
- Women with OUD have demographic differences that include quicker time to physical dependence, shorter duration to adverse outcomes, and higher rates of psychiatric comorbidity.
- Women have improved outcomes rates with care that is trauma-informed, gender-specific, and based in a medical home.
- Treating OUD as a chronic, relapsing, and remitting disease within the concept of a harm-reduction model vastly improves outcomes.

INTRODUCTION

Opioid-use disorder (OUD), which is used interchangeably with the term opioid addiction, has become a societal epidemic with escalating rates in women. It is a chronic illness that does not respect age or sociodemographics. To respond to this epidemic public health crisis, primary care providers need to create the access and workforce training needed to provide the highest quality care possible. Because OUD is a common, chronic disease, it is the duty of primary care providers to lean into learning and treating this condition, and supporting the patients who need assistance.

Disclosure Statement: The authors have nothing to disclose.
Department of Family Medicine, the Larner College of Medicine at the University of Vermont, 235 Rowell, 106 Carrigan Drive, Burlington, VT 05405, USA
* Corresponding author.
E-mail address: Alicia.Jacobs@UVMHealth.org

Prim Care Clin Office Pract 45 (2018) 731–742
https://doi.org/10.1016/j.pop.2018.08.002
0095-4543/18/Published by Elsevier Inc.

primarycare.theclinics.com

EPIDEMIOLOGY
Risk Factors

The biggest risk factors for opioid addiction are adverse childhood events (abuse or trauma), mental health issues, family history of addiction, chronic stress, and chronic pain. In fact, almost all women who develop addiction to opioids have a history of childhood trauma. Psychological and emotional distresses are additional risk factors for women.[1] The United States consumes more than 90% of the opioid pain medications produced in the world and we are 7% of the world's population. Women are generally more likely to have chronic pain complaints. Patients who use pain medications for nonmedical reasons source them predominantly from friends and family, or receives prescription from their own medical provider.[2]

Epidemic Rates

Rates of addiction have skyrocketed in the general population, even more so in women. In 2015 alone, more than 21,500,000 Americans aged 12 years and older were reported to have a substance-use disorder (SUD). Of those, 122,000 were adolescents addicted to prescription pain relievers.[3] At younger ages, there has been full gender convergence so that girls are equally as addicted as boys. Adolescent girls report using to enhance self-esteem, decrease shyness and as a coping skill.[4] The changing burden of disease in women is outlined in **Box 1**.[5]

Complications and Outcomes

There are multiple complications and other health concerns associated with oral and intravenous opioid use, including but not limited to heart or blood stream infections, skin and muscle or bone infections, lung damage, trauma, hepatitis and human immunodeficiency virus, falls, withdrawal symptoms, and concomitant use of other drugs and alcohol. In addition, there are multiple social issues and societal costs, including job loss, family disruption, criminal activity, incarceration, social stigma, loss of housing or custody of children, and an estimated $72 billion in annual health care costs. Women have particularly high rates of multiple providers and emergency department utilization. Rates of hepatitis C more than doubled in the 4 years from 2010 to 2014.[1] Drug overdose killed 52,404 people in 2015, making it the leading cause of accidental death in the United States (**Fig. 1**).[3] Women much more frequently use concomitant benzodiazepines, which markedly increase risk of respiratory depression and death. Incarceration rates are much higher in the United States where drug abuse is predominantly addressed as a criminal behavior in the justice system.[6] Women have a much higher parenting burden and hence expose their own children to adverse childhood

---

Box 1
2015 opioid addiction facts and figures in opioid use disorder in women

- 48,000 died of prescription pain reliever overdose between 1999 and 2010
- Opioid death rates in women have increased by 850% between 1999 and 2015
- Heroin overdose deaths have tripled between 2010 and 2013

Data from American Society of Addiction Medicine. Opioid addiction: 2016 facts & figures. Available at: https://www.asam.org/docs/default-source/advocacy/opioid-addiction-disease-facts-figures.pdf; and Office on Women's Health. Final report: opioid use, misuse, and overdose in women. Available at: https://www.womenshealth.gov/files/documents/final-report-opioid-508.pdf. Accessed December 1, 2017.

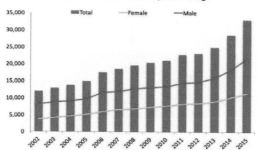

Fig. 1. National overdose deaths. (*From* National Institute on Drug Abuse. Overdose death rate. Available at: https://www.drugabuse.gov/related-topics/trends-statistics/overdose-death-rates; and *Courtesy of* National Center for Health Statistics, CDC Wonder.). Accessed December 1, 2017.

events of addiction, family disruption, and incarceration. This is undoubtedly a public health crisis.

NEUROBIOLOGY

Drug addiction has been defined as the pathologic seeking and using of drugs despite negative consequences.[7] The mechanism is explained by many neurobiological changes to a person's brain causing susceptibility. The most studied is the mesolimbic dopamine system. This system is centered on the nuclear accumbens in the midbrain, with the ventral tegmental area projecting neurons to the forebrain.[8] The areas of forebrain include the hippocampus, amygdala, and prefrontal cortex, which have been implicated as the reward centers of the brain (**Fig. 2**). Although drugs of abuse all are different molecules, their actions all lead to the activation of the mesolimbic dopamine system.[7] Many systems influence and mediate this process, such as gamma-aminobutyric acid (GABA), glutamate, serotonin, and so forth.[9] The stimulation leads to changes in the nerves, which cause them to respond to stimuli differently. Though the paucity of dopamine and other neurotransmitters in these regions rebound with recovery, a relative paucity often remains over time. This accounts for the continued cravings and potential relapses despite years of sobriety.

Many of the early studies on this mesolimbic pathway were conducted in male animal models. In the 1990s, the realization of the importance of the difference between the sexes sparked more research into this area. One of the main areas of study is understanding the effect of estrogen on dopamine. Studies have demonstrated that the subjective effect of cocaine varies based on the menstrual cycle. There is more of a response in the follicular phase when there are relatively high amounts of estrogen and low progesterone. There is much less of an effect in the luteal phase or when subjects have been given high doses of progesterone, indicating progesterone may attenuate the effects of drugs.[10] Estrogen likely plays a role in kappa-opiate binding and mu-opiate binding given that studies have shown increases in premenopausal women compared with men and postmenopausal women.[11] Understanding these differences may help providers in treatment decisions for their patients. For instance, buprenorphine may be a better treatment option for premenopausal women. Inversely, progesterone-only contraception may be a better option for women on opioid replacement.

Women have other differences in their brains that may account for the differences in the timing of onset, severity of addiction, and the telescoping of addiction with faster

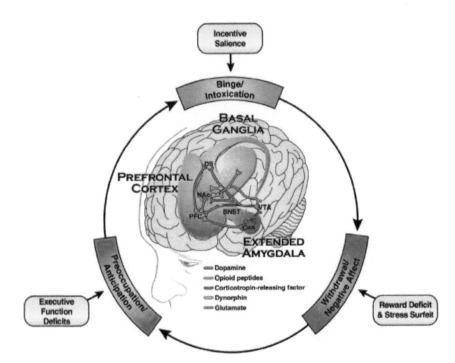

Fig. 2. Anatomy of addiction. CRAFT, car relax alone forget friends trouble. (*Adapted from* Koob GF, Everitt BJ, Robbins TW. Reward, motivation, and addiction. In: Squire LG, Berg D, Bloom FE, et al, editors. Fundamental neuroscience. 3rd edition. Amsterdam: Academic Press; 2008. p. 987–1016; with permission.)

progression of disease. Women have been noted to have more neurons in the ventral tegmental area. Addicting drugs increase dendritic branching of medium spiny neurons, causing more synapses to the reward centers in the forebrain. This is hypothesized to be the reason for women's more rapid progression to drug involvement and dependence.[12]

SCREENING AND DIAGNOSIS

Screening for OUD should be universal, completed with a validated tool, and integrated into standard primary care services. To minimize paperwork fatigue and optimize office workflows, patients should be given a short, evidenced-based, validated tool to assess risk of a SUD. For efficiency, screening can be tiered with a single screening question followed by a confirmatory tool. Eligibility should be based on age rather than demographics and types of visits. The authors recommend screening in the 12 years and older age group at all preventative care visits and other visits as deemed appropriate.

Ideally, questionnaires should be filled out in paper or electronic format directly by the patient because this improves sensitivity rates. In addition, when possible, the tool should be integrated into the usual workflow (integrated into both behavioral health screening and preventative care questionnaires), as well as built into electronic format when applicable.

For the cohort aged 12 to 18 years, the CRAFFT screening tool is recommended. For women 18 years and older, the Single Substance Abuse Question (SSAQ) is a validated primary screening tool recommended by both the National Institute on Drug Abuse (NIDA)[13] and the Substance Abuse and Mental Health Services Association (**Table 1**).[14] Any positive SSAQ screen should be followed with a confirmatory screen. The Drug Abuse Screening Test (DAST)-10 is recommended as an efficient and validated tool (**Table 2**).[15–17] The DAST-10 should be scored and the clinical response should be should matched appropriately with the level of problems related to the drug use. An appropriate response for a low-level score would be brief in office counseling with shorter interval follow-up to reassess risk at a future date. Scores at the moderate to severe level require further investigation and possibly intensive biopsychosocial assessment with an addiction specialist.[18] The continuum of care starts in the primary care office and extends to drug counselor, addiction specialist, and intensive outpatient or inpatient treatment.

TREATMENT: MEDICAL

The Drug Addiction Treatment Act (DATA) was signed in 2000 in response to the increasing prevalence of opioid addiction and heroin overdoses. This effectively allowed for office-based treatment of addiction by allowing physicians to prescribe medications such as buprenorphine. In 2002, the US Food and Drug Administration (FDA) approved 2 formulations of buprenorphine. Pharmacologically, there is no difference between the film and tablet version of buprenorphine. Subjectively, patients seem to prefer the film version of the medication.[19] Buprenorphine works differently than methadone because it is a partial agonist as opposed to a full agonist. Being a partial agonist means that it activates opioid receptors but to a lesser degree than a full agonist. Therefore, people who are used to the subjectively positive effects of opioids will experience a small positive effect, which can increase compliance. It also has a strong affinity to the opioid receptors, which block the effects of full agonists. It still has the potential to be misused but the combination with naloxone minimizes this. Buprenorphine also has a ceiling effect, so increasing the dose of the medication does not produce the same effect as increasing the dose of a full agonist. Buprenorphine is metabolized by cytochrome P450 and, therefore, can have serious drug–drug interactions.[20] Therefore, many sources recommend that buprenorphine should not be used with benzodiazepines or other sedative drugs (eg, alcohol). There is some controversy about whether this is clinically significant versus theoretic risk.

For a physician to begin prescribing, a waiver from the Substance Abuse and Mental Health Service Administration (SAMHSA) must be obtained.[21] To be eligible for this waiver, they must complete an 8-hour training. It is recommended that before beginning to provide office-based addiction treatment services, practices have trained physicians and support staff, as well as connections to mental health resources. In fact, DATA 2000 stipulates that when physicians submit notification to SAMHSA to obtain the required waiver, they must attest to their ability to refer patients for appropriate

Table 1
Screening tool: Single Substance Abuse Question

How many times in the past year have you used an illegal drug or a prescription medication for nonmedical reasons?	None = 0	Once = 1	More than once = 2

From National Institute on Drug Abuse. Resource guide: screening for drug use in general medical settings. Available at: https://www.drugabuse.gov/publications/resource-guide-screening-drug-use-in-general-medical-settings/nida-quick-screen. Accessed December 1, 2017.

Table 2
Screening tool: Drug Abuse Screening Test-10

Drug Use Questionnaire (DAST- 10)		
The following questions concern information about your possible involvement with drugs not including alcoholic beverages during the past 12 mo. Carefully read each statement and decide if your answer is "Yes" or "No". Then, circle the appropriate response beside the question.		
In the statements "drug abuse" refers to (1) the use of prescribed or over the counter drugs may include: cannabis (e.g. marijuana, hash), solvents, tranquillizers (e.g. Valium), barbiturates, cocaine, stimulants (e.g. speed), hallucinogens (e.g. LSD) or narcotics (e.g. heroin). Remember that the questions *do not* include alcoholic beverages.		
Please answer every question. If you have difficulty with a statement, then choose the response that is mostly right.		
These questions refer to the past 12 mo	*Circle Your Response*	
1. Have you used drugs other than those required for medical reasons?	Yes	No
2. Do you abuse more than one drug at a time?	Yes	No
3. Are you always able to stop using drugs when you want to?	Yes	No
4. Have you had "blackouts" or "flashbacks" as a result or drug use?	Yes	No
5. Do you every feel bad or guilty about your drug use?	Yes	No
6. Does your spouse (or parents) ever complain about your involvement with drugs?	Yes	No
7. Have you neglected your family because of your use of drugs?	Yes	No
8. Have you engaged in illegal activities in order to obtain drugs?	Yes	No
9. Have you ever experienced withdrawal symptoms (felt sick) when you stopped taking drugs?	Yes	No
10. Have you had medical problems as a result of your drug use (e.g. memory loss, hepatitis, convulsions, bleeding, etc.)?	Yes	No

© Copyright 1982 by the test author Dr Harvey Skinner, PhD, CPsych, FCAHS, York University, Toronto, Canada and by the Centre for Addiction and Mental Health, Toronto, Canada. Contact the author Dr Skinner at harvey.skinner@yorku.ca regarding permission to use the DAST-10.

counseling and other nonpharmacologic therapy. During the first year, a physician may not treat more than 30 patients. After that time, physicians may request a limit increase to treat no more than 100 patients. Further information on requirements and to find a DATA-approved buprenorphine 8-hour training session can be found on the SAMHSA website. Advanced Practices Providers can also obtain waivers with a 24-hour training.

There are 3 phases to medication-assisted therapy (MAT): induction, stabilization, and maintenance. Induction is the process of switching from the drug of abuse to buprenorphine. The goal is to find the minimum dose at which the patient stops opioid use, has no withdrawal symptoms, has no side effects, and has no cravings. It is recommended that the induction dose or doses be observed, and the patient be followed very closely (1–2 times/week). Stabilization occurs when these criteria have been met. Dosage adjustments may be necessary during early stabilization; however, when the patient reaches maintenance further dose adjustments are not necessary. Frequent contact during stabilization increases likelihood of compliance. It is recommended the patient be seen at least weekly for the first 4 to 5 weeks. The maintenance phase occurs after stabilization and may be indefinite. The visits are spaced out; however, urine drug screening should occur monthly. Because addiction is a relapsing and remitting disease and causes alterations in brain chemistry, patients may need maintenance lifetime treatment. Physicians should be knowledgeable about brief interventions in case of relapse and should give care in a nonjudgmental way. During the maintenance phase, the focus is on psychosocial issues that have been identified during treatment that may contribute to the person's addiction. Many women with SUDs also have a history of trauma. It is important to provide trauma-informed care to these women to reduce the risk of retraumatization and help improve the efficacy of treatment.[22]

TREATMENT: CHRONIC DISEASE, HARM REDUCTION, AND SYSTEMS OF CARE

There has been significant change in the understanding of SUDs over the past few decades. OUD is truly a chronic disease with a relapsing, remitting pattern that includes treatment lapses with nonadherence to recommended treatment, and significant morbidity and mortality. In the past, opioid addiction had been primarily addressed within an abstinence model of care in which treatment was predominantly provided in treatment centers and aimed at complete abstinence from any psychoactive substance use. Any relapse was deemed a failure of treatment.

Understanding the concept of opioid addiction as a chronic disease can help alleviate any perception of treating provider or patient failure. Indeed, when a woman with opioid addiction has a relapse, she is relapsing at a rate comparable to patients with other chronic diseases such as uncontrolled diabetes, hypertension, or asthma (**Fig. 3**).[23] Despite understanding opioid addiction as a chronic disease, many patients and providers still see relapse as a moral failing and shared failure, which can lead to either shame and/or judgment in either party. Relapse in chronic opioid addiction can additionally have more societal impacts due to theft and other crimes. However, the appropriate response to relapse is more targeted wrap-around services rather than discontinuing the doctor and patient relationship.

Understanding opioid addiction as a chronic disease leads to the best outcomes; access to treatment understandably improves outcomes (**Fig. 4**). Using a harm-reduction model of care, access to MAT is ideally made universally available to even further improve outcomes in this epidemic. It is recognized that integrating MAT into the routine, normalized chronic disease management of primary care offices is the ideal mechanism for creating adequate access to care.[24]

Though there could be many models, Vermont uses the hub-and-spoke model, which creates a dynamic movement of patients to and from centralized treatment to decentralized primary care offices, depending on their chronic disease state of

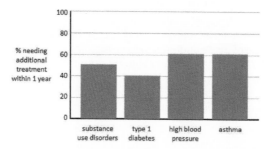

Fig. 3. Relapse rates in chronic medical conditions. (*Data from* McLellan A, Lewis D, O'Brien CP, et al. Drug dependence, a chronic medical illness: implications for treatment, insurance and outcomes evaluation. JAMA 2000;284(13):1689–95.)

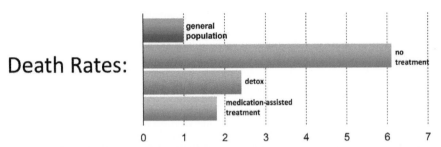

Fig. 4. Outcomes in OUD. (*Data from* Evans E, Li L, Min J, et al. Mortality among individuals accessing pharmacological treatment for opioid dependence in California, 2006-2010. Addiction 2015;110:996–1005; and Mohlman MK, Tanzman B, Finison K, et al. Impact of medication-assisted treatment for opioid addiction on Medicaid expenditures and health services utilization rates in Vermont. J Subst Abuse Treat 2016;67:9–14.)

remission. The hub is the traditional methadone clinic and there are many spokes where patients receive care in ambulatory and other settings. The ideal spoke is the revolutionary, normalized MAT chronic care in the medical home (**Fig. 5**).

Women, in particular, fair less well in the treatment center model of care due to higher rates of parenting responsibilities, more psychiatric comorbidities, and high rates of previous trauma and shame. This centralized model tends to have more associated stigma. In addition, participants can be exposed to supply in the small subset of

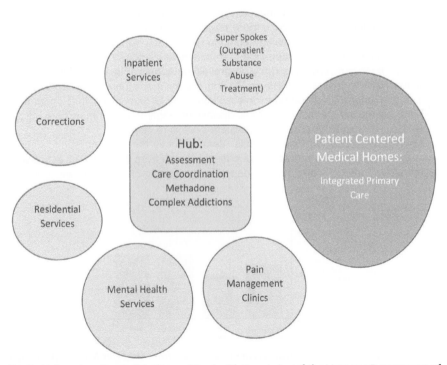

Fig. 5. Hub-and-spoke model of care. (*Used with Permission* of the Vermont Department of Health © 2018.)

relapsing patients in this centralized locations. In a primary care office, appointments can be scheduled around child care, the care is normalized, and psychiatric or other medical concerns can be integrated.

WHOLE PERSON CARE

Working with this high-risk, vulnerable population of women with chronic OUD is a unique opportunity to give whole person care with unconditional regard and a potentially healing relationship. Too often, nonaddiction care is neglected when a patient attends a specialty treatment center. Any of those other health problems, including psychiatric symptoms and untreated medical issues, can affect stress, relapse rates, and overall outcomes. When MAT is provided in a primary care office, it provides a venue of regularly scheduled visits in which other medical and psychiatric care can be provided.

In addition, these more frequent visits provide an opportunity for deeply meaningful connection, which can create an opportunity to provide universal compassion and, therefore, potentially healing relationships. Many of these women have not experienced an unconditional regard to their being and struggles. Validating their struggles, ongoing symptoms of trauma, and right to dignified care is therapeutic for the patient and hence rewarding for the provider to give.

Indeed, in a qualitative study of the Vermont hub-and-spoke model of care, 70% of the participants receiving MAT in the primary care spoke cited the relationship with the doctor as the most important aspect of the location of their care. They also cited access to concomitant medical care, being treated with respect, and being treated without shaming; that is, as a person, not an addict. (Rawson R: Vermont hub-and-spoke model of care for opioid use disorders: An Evaluation. Submitted for publication.) None of the patients receiving care in the centralized hub noted these connections in their treatment center–based care.

SPECIAL CIRCUMSTANCES
Maternity Care

The treatment of drug addiction in pregnancy is a major consideration due to the epidemiology of dependence in women. One-third of all women are in their childbearing years.[25] Both methadone and buprenorphine are approved to treat opioid addiction in nonpregnant patients but both are classified as FDA pregnancy category C medications due to insufficient data regarding their use during pregnancy. It is known that all opioids cross the placental barrier. Prolonged use of any opioids during pregnancy is associated with adverse obstetric outcomes, as well as fetal adverse effects.[26] Neonatal symptoms can include respiratory depression and physical dependence in the neonate and neonatal abstinence syndrome (NAS) shortly after birth. Symptoms of NAS include irritability, hyperactivity, abnormal sleep patterns, failure to gain weight, poor feeding, tremors, vomiting, diarrhea, and high-pitched cry. This condition may become life-threatening without early recognition and treatment.[27] Outcomes in babies are much improved with medically supervised buprenorphine treatment of the gravid mother during pregnancy due to early recognition of NAS symptoms.

Despite the risk of opioid exposure in pregnancy, maternal treatment of OUD during pregnancy is strongly recommended for overall harm reduction. There have been numerous small studies comparing buprenorphine and methadone. One double-blind randomized control study by Jones and colleagues[28] showed no significant difference in the incidence of maternal or neonatal adverse effects. The group treated with buprenorphine had decreased morphine needed to treat NAS and decreased hospital stays. In recent years, buprenorphine has become the standard of care in the treatment of pregnant women.[29] More recently naltrexone has been compared with both buprenorphine and methadone. One study compared naltrexone with buprenorphine, methadone, and nonexposed controls. Results showed that both buprenorphine and naltrexone did not have higher rates of neonatal mortality or congenital abnormalities compared with controls.[30] Based on these early results, providers now have more choice in treatment options for pregnant women. Because buprenorphine monoagent has more potential for abuse and diversion, many centers are now using buprenorphine or naloxone for MAT therapy in pregnant women.

Dental

Any person on long-term opioids is at higher risk for dental caries, periodontal disease, and tooth loss, which can lead to taste impairment and eating difficulties. The reasons behind this increased risk of oral health problems may be multifactorial, including poor oral hygiene, chronic pain, and xerostomia from salivary hypofunction (from the medications). All patients on MAT should have an assessment of their oral health and be connected with a dental home.[31]

Tobacco

Tobacco use is 4 times higher in patients with opioid abuse history than the general population. Tobacco abuse is a high-prevalence preventable cause of morbidity and mortality in the United States. In fact, the prevalence of smoking in patients with SUDs exceeds 70%.[18] Although nicotine triggers the same pleasure pathways in the brain as opioids, medications used to treat opioid dependence do not seem to have a significant effect on smoking cessation.[32] These patients also tend to minimize the importance of cigarette smoking in their overall health.[33] Due to frequency of visits for MAT, there is ample opportunity to address tobacco use in this population. Likewise, because smoking can cause serious complications in pregnancy, this is an important time to address smoking cessation.

Other Comorbidities

More than 60% of patients with SUD have coexisting psychiatric illness, including mood, anxiety, psychotic, attention-deficit hyperactivity, and antisocial personality disorders. In addition, other drug use, posttraumatic stress disorder, unwanted pregnancies, eating disorders, and premenstrual dysphoric disorder occur at higher rates.

Lapses in Care

Of note, many patients experience lapses in insurance coverage and hence coverage of their care that puts them at increased risk for relapse. Inversely, relapse can put these patients at increased risk for neglect of maintaining their insurance coverage.

SUMMARY

Societally, the deadly epidemic of OUD is skyrocketing in women, causing increasing disease burden and fatalities. Primary care clinicians must consider the top reasons to provide integrated management of opioid addiction in women in the primary care office:

1. Opioid addiction is epidemic and rates are rising even faster in women.
2. Treating the addiction with MAT vastly improves outcomes, particularly in women who have disproportionate parenting responsibilities.

3. Providing MAT in primary care normalizes the care and reduces shame.
4. Providing MAT in primary care creates the opportunity for whole person care, including every psychiatric and medical problem.
5. Women with OUD are a vulnerable population and each person needs a champion.
6. Providing this type of integrated care creates the opportunity for primary care practice to be inspired, inspirational, and unconditional.

ACKNOWLEDGMENTS

Many thanks to Drs Patricia Fisher and Sanchit Maruti for their expert input into this article, and to Dr Michael Goedde for statistics and figures.

REFERENCES

1. Final Report: Opioid use, Misues and Overdose in Women. 2017. Available at: https://www.womenshealth.gov/files/documents/final-report-opioid-508.pdf. Accessed December 1, 2017.
2. Jones C, Paulozzi L, Mack K. Sources of Prescription opioid pain relievers by frequency of past year non-medical use: United States, 2008-2011. JAMA 2014; 174(5):802–3.
3. A. S. o. A. Medicine. 2016. Available at: http://www.asam.org/docs/default-source/advocacy/opioid-addiction-disease-facts-figures.pdf. Accessed December 1, 2017.
4. Zilberman M. Substance abuse across the lifespan in women, in Women & Addiction. The Guilford Press; 2009. p. 3–13.
5. Opioid Addiction Facts & Figures 2016, American Society of Addiction Medicine. Available: https://www.asam.org/docs/default-source/advocacy/opioid-addiction-disease-facts-figures.pdf. Accessed December 1, 2017.
6. Hser Y, Evans E, Grella C, et al. Long-term course of opioid addiction. Harv Rev Psychiatry 2014;23(2):76–89.
7. Hyman SE. Addiction: a disease of learning and memory. Am J Psychiatry 2005; 162:1414–22.
8. Nestler EJ. Cellular basis of memory for addiction. Dialogues Clin Neurosci 2013; 15:431–43.
9. Nestler EJ. Molecular basis of long-term plasticity underlying addiction. Nat Rev Neurosci 2001;2:119–28.
10. Evans SM, Foltin RW. Exogenous progesterone attenuates the subjective effects of smoked cocaine in women, but not in men. Neuropsychopharmacology 2006; 31:659–74.
11. Zubieta J-K, Dannals RF, Frost J. Gender and age influences on human brain mu-opioid receptor binding measured by PET. Am J Psychiatry 1999;156:842–8.
12. Bobzean S, DeNorbrega A, Perrotti L. Sex differences in the neurobiology of drug addiction. Exp Neurol 2014;259:64–74.
13. National Institute on Drug Abuse. Available at: https://www.drugabuse.gov/publications/resource-guide-screening-drug-use-in-general-medical-settings/nida-quick-screen. Accessed December 1, 2017.
14. Substance Abuse and Mental Health Services Association. Available at: https://www.samhsa.gov/. Accessed December 1, 2017.
15. Yudko E, Lozhkina O, Fouts A. A comprehensive review of the psychometric properties of the Drug Abuse Screening Test. J Subst Abuse Treat 2007;32: 189–98.

16. Gavin D, Ross H, Skinner H. Diagnostic validity of the Drug Abuse Screening Test in the assessment of DSM-III drug disorders. Br J Addict 1989;84(3):301–7.

17. Skinner HA. The Drug Abuse Screening Test. Addict Behav 1982;7(4):363–71.

18. LaPaglia D. Substance use disorders and systems of care. In: Yale textbook of public psychiatry. Oxford University Press; 2016. p. 81–96.

19. Soyka M. Buprenorphine-naloxone buccal soluble film for the treatment of opioid dependence: current update. Expert Opin Drug Deliv 2015;12(2):339–47.

20. Johnson R, Strain E, Amass L. Buprenorphine: how to use it right. Drug Alcohol Depend 2003;70:59–77.

21. Samhsa, Samhsa. 2016. Available at: https://www.samhsa.gov/medication-assisted-treatment/buprenorphine-waiver-management/. Accessed November 30, 2017.

22. Brown V, Harris M, Fallot R. Moving toward trauma-informed practice in addiction treatment: a collaborative model of agency assessment. J Psychoactive Drugs 2013;45(5):386–93.

23. McLellan AT, Lewis DC, O'Brien CP, et al. Drug dependence, a chronic medical illness: implications for treatment, insurance, and outcomes evaluation. JAMA 2000;284:1689–95.

24. Brooklyn J, Sigmon S. Vermont hub-and-spoke model of care for opioid use disorder: development, implementation, and impact. J Addict Med 2017;11:286–92.

25. Unger A, Jung E, Winklbaur B, et al. Gender issues in the pharmacotherapy of opioid-addicted women: buprenorphine. J Addict Dis 2010;29:217–30.

26. Ludlow JP, Evans SF, Hulse G. Obstetric and perinatal outcomes in pregnancies associated with illicit substance abuse. Aust N Z J Obstet Gynaecol 2004;44:302–6.

27. Oei J, Lui K. Managment of the newborn infant affected by maternal opiates and other drugs of dependency. J Paediatr Child Health 2007;43:9–18.

28. Jones HE, Kaltenbach K, Heil SH, et al. Neonatal abstinence syndrome after methadone or buprenorphine exposure. N Engl J Med 2010;363:2320–31.

29. Soyka M. Buprenorphine use in pregnant opioid users: a critical review. CNS Drugs 2013;27(8):653–62.

30. Kelty E, Hulse G. A retrospective cohort study of obstetric outcomes in opioid-dependent women treated with implant naltrexone, oral methadone or sublingual buprenorphine, and non-dependent controls. Drugs 2017;77:1199–210.

31. Shekarchizadeh H, Khami MR, Mohebbi SZ. Oral health of drug abusers: a review of health effects and care. Iran J Public Health 2013;42(9):929–40.

32. David SP, Lancaster T, Stead L, et al. Opioid antagonists for smoking cessation. Cochrane Database Syst Rev 2013;(6):CD003086.

33. Mandal P, Jain R, Jhanjee S, et al. Psychological barriers to tobacco cessation in Indian buprenorphine-naloxone maintained patients: a pilot study. Indian J Psychol Med 2015;37:299–304.

UNITED STATES POSTAL SERVICE ® Statement of Ownership, Management, and Circulation (All Periodicals Publications Except Requester Publications)

1. Publication Title	2. Publication Number	3. Filing Date
PRIMARY CARE: CLINICS IN OFFICE PRACTICE	044 – 690	9/18/2018

4. Issue Frequency	5. Number of Issues Published Annually	6. Annual Subscription Price
MAR, JUN, SEP, DEC	4	$237.00

7. Complete Mailing Address of Known Office of Publication (Not printer) (Street, city, county, state, and ZIP+4®)

ELSEVIER INC.
230 Park Avenue, Suite 800
New York, NY 10169

Contact Person
STEPHEN R. BUSHING

Telephone (Include area code)
215-239-3688

8. Complete Mailing Address of Headquarters or General Business Office of Publisher (Not printer)

ELSEVIER INC.
230 Park Avenue, Suite 800
New York, NY 10169

9. Full Names and Complete Mailing Addresses of Publisher, Editor, and Managing Editor (Do not leave blank)

Publisher (Name and complete mailing address)

TAYLOR E BALL, ELSEVIER INC.
1600 JOHN F KENNEDY BLVD. SUITE 1800
PHILADELPHIA, PA 19103-2899

Editor (Name and complete mailing address)

JESSICA MCCOOL, ELSEVIER INC.
1600 JOHN F KENNEDY BLVD. SUITE 1800
PHILADELPHIA, PA 19103-2899

Managing Editor (Name and complete mailing address)

PATRICK MANLEY, ELSEVIER INC.
1600 JOHN F KENNEDY BLVD. SUITE 1800
PHILADELPHIA, PA 19103-2899

10. Owner (Do not leave blank. If the publication is owned by a corporation, give the name and address of the corporation immediately followed by the names and addresses of all stockholders owning or holding 1 percent or more of the total amount of stock. If not owned by a corporation, give the names and addresses of the individual owners. If owned by a partnership or other unincorporated firm, give its name and address as well as those of each individual owner. If the publication is published by a nonprofit organization, give its name and address.)

Full Name	Complete Mailing Address
WHOLLY OWNED SUBSIDIARY OF REED/ELSEVIER, US HOLDINGS	1600 JOHN F KENNEDY BLVD. SUITE 1800 PHILADELPHIA, PA 19103-2899

11. Known Bondholders, Mortgagees, and Other Security Holders Owning or Holding 1 Percent or More of Total Amount of Bonds, Mortgages, or Other Securities. If none, check box → ☐ None

Full Name	Complete Mailing Address
N/A	

12. Tax Status (For completion by nonprofit organizations authorized to mail at nonprofit rates) (Check one)
The purpose, function, and nonprofit status of this organization and the exempt status for federal income tax purposes:
☒ Has Not Changed During Preceding 12 Months
☐ Has Changed During Preceding 12 Months (Publisher must submit explanation of change with this statement)

PS Form 3526, July 2014 [Page 1 of 4 (see instructions page 4)]   PSN: 7530-01-000-9931   PRIVACY NOTICE: See our privacy policy on www.usps.com.

13. Publication Title		14. Issue Date for Circulation Data Below
PRIMARY CARE: CLINICS IN OFFICE PRACTICE		JUNE 2018

15. Extent and Nature of Circulation			Average No. Copies Each Issue During Preceding 12 Months	No. Copies of Single Issue Published Nearest to Filing Date
a. Total Number of Copies (Net press run)			98	133
b. Paid Circulation (By Mail and Outside the Mail)	(1)	Mailed Outside-County Paid Subscriptions Stated on PS Form 3541 (Include paid distribution above nominal rate, advertiser's proof copies, and exchange copies)	42	47
	(2)	Mailed In-County Paid Subscriptions Stated on PS Form 3541 (Include paid distribution above nominal rate, advertiser's proof copies, and exchange copies)	0	0
	(3)	Paid Distribution Outside the Mails Including Sales Through Dealers and Carriers, Street Vendors, Counter Sales, and Other Paid Distribution Outside USPS®	12	16
	(4)	Paid Distribution by Other Classes of Mail Through the USPS (e.g., First-Class Mail®)	0	0
c. Total Paid Distribution (Sum of 15b (1), (2), (3), and (4))			54	63
d. Free or Nominal Rate Distribution (By Mail and Outside the Mail)	(1)	Free or Nominal Rate Outside-County Copies Included on PS Form 3541	29	54
	(2)	Free or Nominal Rate In-County Copies Included on PS Form 3541	0	0
	(3)	Free or Nominal Rate Copies Mailed at Other Classes Through the USPS (e.g., First-Class Mail)	0	0
	(4)	Free or Nominal Rate Distribution Outside the Mail (Carriers or other means)	0	0
e. Total Free or Nominal Rate Distribution (Sum of 15d (1), (2), (3) and (4))			29	54
f. Total Distribution (Sum of 15c and 15e)			83	117
g. Copies not Distributed (See Instructions to Publishers #4 (page #3))			15	16
h. Total (Sum of 15f and g)			98	133
i. Percent Paid (15c divided by 15f times 100)			65.06%	53.85%

* If you are claiming electronic copies, go to line 16 on page 3. If you are not claiming electronic copies, skip to line 17 on page 3.

16. Electronic Copy Circulation		Average No. Copies Each Issue During Preceding 12 Months	No. Copies of Single Issue Published Nearest to Filing Date
a. Paid Electronic Copies	▲	0	0
b. Total Paid Print Copies (Line 15c) + Paid Electronic Copies (Line 16a)	▲	54	63
c. Total Print Distribution (Line 15f) + Paid Electronic Copies (Line 16a)	▲	83	117
d. Percent Paid (Both Print & Electronic Copies) (16b divided by 16c × 100)		65.06%	53.85%

☒ I certify that 50% of all my distributed copies (electronic and print) are paid above a nominal price.

17. Publication of Statement of Ownership

☒ If the publication is a general publication, publication of this statement is required. Will be printed
in the DECEMBER 2018 issue of this publication.

☐ Publication not required.

18. Signature and Title of Editor, Publisher, Business Manager, or Owner

[signature]   Date 9/18/2018

STEPHEN R. BUSHING - INVENTORY DISTRIBUTION CONTROL MANAGER

I certify that all information furnished on this form is true and complete. I understand that anyone who furnishes false or misleading information on this form or who omits material or information requested on the form may be subject to criminal sanctions (including fines and imprisonment) and/or civil sanctions (including civil penalties).

PS Form 3526, July 2014 (Page 3 of 4)   PRIVACY NOTICE: See our privacy policy on www.usps.com.

Moving?

Make sure your subscription moves with you!

To notify us of your new address, find your **Clinics Account Number** (located on your mailing label above your name), and contact customer service at:

Email: journalscustomerservice-usa@elsevier.com

800-654-2452 (subscribers in the U.S. & Canada)
314-447-8871 (subscribers outside of the U.S. & Canada)

Fax number: 314-447-8029

Elsevier Health Sciences Division
Subscription Customer Service
3251 Riverport Lane
Maryland Heights, MO 63043

*To ensure uninterrupted delivery of your subscription, please notify us at least 4 weeks in advance of move.

Printed and bound by CPI Group (UK) Ltd, Croydon, CR0 4YY

03/10/2024

01040391-0015